BETTER POSTURE FAST

How to Finally End Chronic Neck and Back Pain

Philip V. Cordova, D.C. &
Natalie A. Cordova, D.C.

iUniverse®

BETTER POSTURE FAST
HOW TO FINALLY END CHRONIC NECK AND BACK PAIN

iUniverse books may be ordered through booksellers or by contacting:

iUniverse
1663 Liberty Drive
Bloomington, IN 47403
www.iuniverse.com
844-349-9409

ISBN: 978-1-6632-3040-9 (sc)
ISBN: 978-1-6632-3087-4 (e)

Library of Congress Control Number: 2021921684

Print information available on the last page.

iUniverse rev. date: 11/12/2021

With contributions from:
Kevin Wafer, D.C.
Brandon Siegmund, D.C.
Bryen Brown, D.C.
Michael Cooper, D.C.
Jesse West, D.C.

CONTENTS

INTRODUCTION

Millions of people suffer daily with chronic neck and back pain. We meet these patients every day in our chiropractic office, and so many of them have no idea why they hurt or what caused their symptoms to begin.

They tell us things like:

- ➲ "I didn't even do anything – it just started hurting."
- ➲ "Maybe I slept wrong?"
- ➲ "I turned my head to check my blind spot, and it just stayed like this."
- ➲ "I bent down to pick up a pair of socks from the floor, and I couldn't get back up."

Some patients have just given up on the idea that anything can be done about it. "I know that if something falls on the floor, it's just going to stay there. There's no way I'm going to be able to pick it up." They've given up on exercising or enjoying many of the activities they've done for years because the pain just isn't worth it or because they can't move like they used to. Their daily activities just aren't fun anymore.

Some patients don't realize how bad they've gotten. We'll do an examination and find that they can turn their head only about half as far as they should be able to do. The pain they used to have has lessened (*or gone away completely*), so they believe the problem has resolved. Or they'll come in for a low-back problem, unaware that their neck has terribly limited range of motion.

Then, if we take X-rays, they're shocked by the level of degeneration already present in their spine. They'll ask, "Everyone has this, right?" or maybe they'll say, "It's because I'm getting older, right?" We hear the "older" comment from patients in their twenties and all the way up. (*We also see people of all ages with great spines too, so it's not all about age.*) Do you know how hard it is to explain to a twenty-five-year-old that they're not old yet – even though their spine shows aging beyond their years?

How does it happen? How do people end up in pain with advanced degenerative changes without already realizing they had a problem?

People get spinal degeneration one of two ways. The first is due to some sort of a trauma, whether it happened recently or sometime way in the past. They've been in a car accident, fallen down, or suffered an accident a while ago when playing with friends ("*It didn't seem like a big deal at the time*"), and they realize they've never been the same. While we usually remember the big traumas in our life (*e.g., "I never fully recovered after that last car accident," or "I crashed my bike, and my low back just never got back to how it was before*"), your life has been filled with traumas you've overlooked.

The other cause of spinal degeneration relates to your daily activities – the little, often overlooked, imbalanced daily activities that would never cause a problem when done just once ... little things you do all the time without considering how it may affect your spine. When we do that activity over and over again on a daily basis, and that daily basis turns into weeks and months ... well, it adds up.

These are the activities that cause the problems slowly over time and leave you believing that you "didn't do anything" to cause the problem. These are the activities that build up until your spine can't take it anymore and then – BAM! You've got a symptom. The truth is you're always doing *something*. Some things are good for your neck and back, while other things are not so good. Rarely is anything neutral. Gravity is a constant force that we battle daily to resist and how we resist gravity plays a big part in how our spine ages.

The way you resist gravity, the extent to which your activities are balanced, and the degree to which you work to overcome any imbalances are going to combine to be your winning formula to avoid chronic neck and back pain. Our goal for this book is to make you aware of the things you're doing to lead to these problems, to teach you how to overcome them on your own, and to share what you can do if you can't do it on your own.

In the last twenty-five years of treating patients, we have found that many of the issues that cause a patient to enter a chiropractic office are caused by the same problem. All of the mysterious pains that seem to "suddenly show up out of nowhere" can almost always be linked to the same cause. While most people are puzzled when they come in for their initial consultation, we can take one look at how they sit in the waiting room or how they walk and know exactly what's needed to get them feeling better and keep the symptoms from coming back.

They're going to have to work on improving their posture.

Whether they'll listen to us is another story altogether. It's not that they don't believe working on their posture will reduce their pain and improve their health; they just hope there's another way to go about it. People are used to taking a pill to make them feel better, or they look for a "miracle" to fix their problem. They're busy, and they don't want to add one more thing to their to-do list, especially if they have even a small doubt about the expected results. (*We occasionally have patients who have heard a story about someone going to see a chiropractor who got "cracked" once and then never had that problem again: "My friend just got cracked, and he didn't have to do any exercises. Why should I?"*)

They want something that doesn't require any work on their part to make it happen, but that's not very realistic. We encourage our patients to participate in their recovery and their results. We love patients that seek chiropractic care for a lifetime, but feel our best patients do not seek dependence on our care. Rather, they want to take an active role in their own health. There are plenty of reasons to get your spine adjusted that have nothing to do with relieving pain. Better posture and the right exercises can help your spine stay strong. This means we will need your participation! We guide our patients on the steps to take to be successful, but patients still have to do their part to create a lasting change.

When we asked one of our first patients about doing some of the home exercises we recommended for her, she stated matter-of-factly, "You're doing great on your own, Doc." This meant that she was getting adjusted and seeing results, so she didn't do a single home recommendation that would keep the problem from coming back. She didn't see any reason to do anything more than show up to our office because everything seemed to be working great. We love to see our patients get better, but we still think you can help to make it a long-lasting change.

Our first patients came to see us before there were smartphones and before everyone spent so much time in front of a computer every day. Most of the bad-posture habits we saw back then came from sitting at a desk, driving, and slouching on a couch at home. At that time, patients didn't have their heads tilted straight down, looking at their phones all day.

Now people spend nearly all day in bad posture, and some continue that process at night, slouching on their couch and then sleeping in a bad postural position. We see people standing in line, staring down at their phones in what is easily the world's worst neck position and we wonder how they can live like that. Then they come to see us for a follow-up visit and mention that their neck and back still hurt: "I feel great when I leave and for a couple days after, but then the pain comes back."

Shocking! (*Kidding, this is not shocking.*)

Even if every patient spent thirty minutes in our office every single day (*no one does this*), they would still be responsible for doing good things for their spine for twenty-three and a half hours a day. Unfortunately, they are more likely to do bad things that can make them worse. Since people spend so much time causing problems for their spine, it's truly amazing that they don't have more neck and back pain.

Bad posture can be changed, but most people go about making that change the wrong way. They don't understand the basics of how it got that bad and what they're doing to continue to make it worse. Some people attempt to improve their posture, but they don't do enough to change quickly. Slow progress means they don't feel like what they're doing is worth it, so they give up.

That's about to change.

We are going to explain how to make fast changes to your bad posture. We believe if you can start to see changes in how you look and how you feel about yourself, and if you can decrease your pain quickly, you'll know this will work. And if it's working, hopefully you'll keep it up. This is how you can finally end your chronic neck and back pain and keep it from coming back.

Some patients do great at first, then go back to their old habits. After reading this book, you won't be one of those people, right? You'll know what to do to relieve the pain and get back to good posture in record time. This book is about changing how you approach your neck and back pain so you can minimize the time you're not feeling as good as you should.

This book is the result of more than two decades of seeing and helping people get better. We've had some time to see what people will actually do to make changes, and what is just too much to ask an average person to get done on a daily basis.

Most of us know many of the right things to do, but we don't do them because there are so many other things to do. Our patients tend to be busy people, so this book will help you zero in on the fastest route to making changes to your posture without turning it into a full-time job.

You'll also learn how we do things in our office. While not completely unique in our process, we've found that our process is not common across the board for all chiropractors. We're going to show you how to make changes to your posture as much as you can without our help. When you do need our help, you'll understand why our process and treatment plans get such great results.

We can't wait to see how better posture helps you lead a healthier and pain-free life. Let's get started!

A TYPICAL
POSTURE STORY

Susan works at a computer all day and regularly has neck and back pain. About once a week, she also experiences a headache at the back of her head. The neck and back pain usually goes away with some rubbing of the muscles and a little ibuprofen. A combination of massaging and other over-the-counter medications knocks out the associated headache at the back of her head in a day or two.

Lately, though, she's noticed a "hump" forming on her upper back. She feels like it sticks out and thinks everyone must be staring at it. Embarrassed by her developing hump, she's started to avoid wearing clothes that leave the area exposed for all to see. When she goes to the internet to determine what she can do about it, that just scares her more. She reads a webpage that describes the "Dowager's hump" – a permanent, painful condition largely due to osteoporosis. She is just thirty years old. She couldn't have osteoporosis already … could she?

She goes to her family doctor, has a bone density test, and gets her results. "Your bone density is fine," says her MD. "You don't have osteoporosis. It may be time to start working on your posture. Just try to remember to sit up straight more often."

Determined to make a change, she puts sticky notes up around her office and even buys a gadget that hooks to her shirt and buzzes every time she slouches. This becomes annoying very quickly. She hadn't realized how much she slouches, but staying upright throughout the day is proving to be quite the challenge.

Her social media feed shows her an ad for a posture brace that will hold her shoulders back in the right position all day. She places her order, and a week later receives her brace. The brace feels great at first. Is this what good posture is supposed to feel like? She's happy with how she looks in the mirror and is grateful to have found the answer. She'll wear this brace every day and finally have good posture! Or will she?

After a few weeks of wearing the brace, she decides to take a break. It's become tedious to put on a brace just to get some work done, and it isn't helping as much as it once did. Not wearing the brace for just a day leads to a lot of neck and upper back pain. She hadn't realized that the longer you wear a brace, the weaker your muscles become. She's become dependent on the brace!

Now she finds herself wearing the brace, but it doesn't feel as good as it did in the beginning. Her neck and back continue to be a problem, and her headaches are more intense and more frequent. She's taking pain relievers now just to get her work done.

Frustrated, she tells her friends and co-workers all about it. One of her friends happens to be our patient and mentions how focused we are on helping people with chronic neck and back pain, especially when it may be due to a posture problem.

Susan comes into our office, and we start with a consultation, examination, and X-rays of her spine. We review her examination and take a series of measurements on her X-rays to establish a starting point and show her exactly how much her spine needs to change. (*This will also give us an idea of how much she has improved when we do follow-up X-rays down the road.*)

We show her that her spine has early signs of degeneration in her neck and upper back. We can see the "hump" that worries her, but the X-rays make it clear that the changes are not yet permanent. There is some work to do, but it is manageable.

We give her guidance on how to set up her workstation in a more posture-friendly way and start her on a personalized chiropractic care program. She receives specific spinal adjustments that are guided by the measurements we did on her X-rays. Finally, she receives at-home posture recommendations aimed at improving her neck curve. Additionally, we provide posture exercises and stretches that will help the improvements stay in place a lot longer.

For a few months, she is diligent and consistent with the recommendations. We take a few follow-up X-rays and remeasure the curves and disc spaces that we typically do as part of our analysis. Her curve has improved significantly, and she is making long-term structural improvements.

Susan took action earlier in her life than most people do and was able to see a change. Unfortunately, the average first-time chiropractic patient is approximately forty-five years old, and a lot of permanent changes have occurred by then.

Have you ever been embarrassed by your bad posture? Have you looked at a photo and thought, "Well, that doesn't look good"? Are you worried about developing a "hump"? Have you already started to experience symptoms like headaches, neck pain, or back pain due to your poor posture?

Susan's bad-posture journey may sound familiar to your story because it certainly sounds familiar to us. While "Susan's" story is an example, it's one we've heard many times. Everyone starts with the same idea: trying to remember to have better posture before moving on to an assortment of posture supports or gadgets.

In this example, Susan stopped trying to figure it out on her own after just one gadget and posture brace. In reality, patients often spend a lot of money on various products before they finally throw up their hands and come to us. They may even try working out to change things, but since they don't do enough of the right exercises and stretches, they rarely see a difference. Even worse, they are wasting valuable time to make changes to their spine. From the initial awareness of the problem to actually taking the right action, the person may wait years.

Sometimes vertebrae are just out of place and no longer working like they should. This can make improving your posture more of a challenge than you think it should be. There's really no way for you to know how long it will take or the extent to which your posture has affected your neck and your spine without an evaluation, but you can still see significant changes when you start doing the right things and stop doing the wrong things.

This book contains everything you need to know to change your posture fast (*so you can feel better*), but it also includes guidance on how to maintain the good posture you achieved (*so you can keep feeling better*).

If you take consistent action, you will get better posture fast. What difference would changing your posture make in your life? How differently will you feel about yourself when you're standing tall, free of pain? While reading this book, you need to keep your goal in mind. Finding the "why" behind your goal to have better posture will significantly increase the likelihood that you will hit your target.

Our goal in writing this book is to give you actionable steps to make a change. If you start doing research on improving your posture, you'll see images of the exact angles where your head and neck should be when sitting at a computer (*e.g., are your elbows at the perfect angle?*). That type of information is not what you'll get in this book. We've yet to see a patient take the time to measure their wrist angle to see if they're ergonomically correct. Instead, we'll teach you some common-sense approaches and some rules of thumb so you can see changes without driving yourself crazy.

Because there are tons of posture braces, supports, gadgets, exercises, and stretches out there, you'll get information overload searching the internet for "help for better posture." Let us help you get what you need to make the greatest improvement in the shortest amount of time and, hopefully, help you save time and money you would have wasted on the wrong things. Your posture needs to change now – there's no time to waste on the wrong stuff!

While we may give you more information than you may want at

this exact moment, this book is filled with the answers to questions our patients commonly ask. You may not care about choosing the right desk chair today, but you'll still find information about it here. You may not be interested in how to save your neck on a long car trip, but we'll tell you about it anyway. You may not be ready for some of the more challenging exercises, but they'll be here when you hit that level.

We've also included tips, strategies, and exercises for all age levels and abilities. Maybe you've started to notice your upper back is looking more like your grandmother's than you would like and you're ready to change. If you're already a very fit person, we think you'll still find some worthwhile strategies regarding how you set up your computer, what to stretch, and some targeted exercises that will make all the difference.

A few benefits of good posture that can be experienced almost immediately include:

- ⮂ Appearing more confident
- ⮂ Being taller
- ⮂ Breathing easier
- ⮂ Reducing stress
- ⮂ Stopping headaches
- ⮂ Decreasing neck and back pain
- ⮂ Eliminating the "burning pain" between shoulder blades
- ⮂ Moving better

Some long-term benefits of better posture include the following:

- ⮂ Avoiding "the hump"
- ⮂ Lessening the severity of any "hump" that may be forming
- ⮂ Maintaining the health of spinal discs
- ⮂ Avoiding complications of osteoporosis
- ⮂ Avoiding degenerative conditions of the spine
- ⮂ Being able to keep moving and staying active without pain

We've worked with patients with a multitude of neck, back, hip, and shoulder problems that can all be directly linked to their bad-posture habits. We see younger patients with advanced degrees of spinal degeneration and elderly patients with the spines of someone half their age.

We regularly take spinal X-rays in our clinic and have seen many in which the age of the patient doesn't match what's on the film (*good and bad*). We have to double-check to make sure we are looking at the right X-rays! More and more often, we are seeing the damage caused by bad posture on X-rays, including changes to the structures of the bones, degeneration, and even a "horn" that can grow from the base of the skull due to long-term forward head posture. There's no hiding bad-posture damage on an X-ray.

Occasionally, we see healthy, normal X-rays in patients that are advanced in age. When we see this, it's due to healthy habits and activities that have been part of what they have done on a regular basis throughout their lives. They've developed good posture habits without specifically trying to work on their posture, and it worked!

Our mindset and approach to achieving good posture is this: Let's make the tweaks to your activities that are causing the most damage, give you the right stretches and exercises that will make the greatest difference, get your spine in the right alignment with chiropractic care, recommend products that will actually help, and give you things to do that will help you keep that improved posture.

This book was created after answering our patients' questions and seeing their concerns for twenty-five years. We want our patients to have a resource when they need posture information. When we checked out what was available, we found the available information to be too technical, too complicated, or a thinly veiled attempt to sell you a device or gadget.

This book is here to help you change your posture for good. Are you ready to enjoy better posture? Are you ready to be healthier? We'll show you how to make a change to your posture without spending any money. You certainly can spend money on products and services that will help accelerate results, so we will offer suggestions and recommendations for additional products and services that we believe in.

The solution to your posture problem doesn't need to be complicated; it just needs to get done. Remember, it's most often your simple, uncomplicated daily activities and movements that have resulted in your current posture. It's simple changes to daily activities over time that will change that posture for good.

▶ CHAPTER 1

HOW YOUR POSTURE FORMS

Have you ever thought about how your posture forms in the first place? Your body is designed to work a specific way, and to work well. It makes sense that the natural curves of your spine are there for a specific purpose.

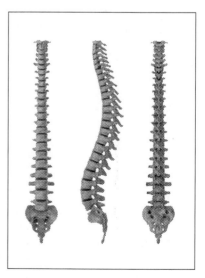

When viewed from the side, your spine is supposed to have three curves. Your neck and low back curve the same way, in what's called a lordotic curve. Your mid-back curves the other way (*sometimes too much*), and this is called a kyphotic curve.

These are your normal curves, the ones you're supposed to have. When your spine has these curves in their ideal degrees, it's at its strongest. Additionally, from the side view, your ears should line up with your shoulders and your shoulders should line up with your hips. Maintaining these curves and keeping your body parts where they are supposed to be are important for good posture, but even more important for good health.

As chiropractors, we continually educate our patients on the importance of the spine as it relates to the spinal cord and nerves. The nervous system is the first system that forms and is literally the "life force" that makes your body work and function. The technology exists to replace your heart, lungs, liver, etc., and still survive and thrive. However, there's no replacement for your spine or your nerves. Caring for your spine is caring for your nervous system. That's why we focus so much on your spine's positioning, movement, and health.

In a discussion with a dentist about our respective areas of focus, we reminded him, "You can get new teeth, but you can't get a new spine." Even so, most people brush, floss, whiten, and regularly see their dentist to make sure their smile is as good as it can be. Only about 10 percent of the population regularly see a chiropractor. When asked, as many as 66 percent of people polled said they would consider visiting a chiropractor, but the real numbers are nowhere close to that.

Because we can't see our spine or watch the damage as it occurs, we don't take the health of our spine and nervous system as seriously as we do our teeth. Better posture and good spinal health are not just about preventing or relieving pain. They can literally extend your life, and most definitely increase the quality of your life.

When you're born, you have only one spinal curve. Your neck, mid-back, and low back all have the same kyphotic curve. Picture the fetal position, and you'll see what we mean by the kyphotic curve. This is the position you're in when you're still in the womb. Unfortunately, bad posture will move you back to this position if you're not careful.

At first, having just one curve is fine because you're not doing a lot of activities that require you to resist gravity. Basically, you're just being carried around. Your first "big moment" is when you're finally able to hold up your head on your own. That's when you begin to develop your neck curve, called a lordotic curve.

With this first lordotic curve, your neck muscles begin to determine what your neck posture will be for years to come. As you practice holding up your head, you go from shaking and awkward until it becomes a natural part of how you move. Your neck gets stronger, and it's able to support your head normally and comfortably.

The next phase is when you start crawling, which reinforces your neck strength and initiates the development of the lordotic curve in your lower back. Next, you begin standing, and then walking. With walking, you experience a full upright position and activities that require you to resist gravity. The curves all begin to stabilize as your body gains muscle control and strength. Rushing through any of these stages may affect posture early on. We have to build up the strength at each stage to have the right posture.

If it's in alignment and has all the right curves, your spine will be the strongest it can be. When the spine becomes misaligned or loses any of its curves, it becomes weaker and more susceptible to pain and problems – like neck and back pain.

If your spinal curves all form based on using your muscles and teaching your spine to stay a certain way, then it follows that the way you continue to use your muscles will determine how your spine changes throughout your life. This is why hunching over a computer or slouching begins to alter the curves you initially developed.

This is also why giving a toddler a tablet and allowing them to look down at the device for hours on end will change the development of the curve of their neck. Having a tablet isn't the problem – it's the position they stay in for extended periods. (*This is probably why we see more kids that already have the bad posture that took their parents many years to develop.*) Your problem isn't your computer – it's how you sit while using it.

The same muscles that created your posture in the first place will determine how good your posture will become and how well you'll be able to maintain your results. Almost any activity you want to do can be done with good or bad posture. Whichever position or movement you do the most is the most likely to win.

We're initially set up to have good posture, given the way our body starts to develop. It's the accidents, injuries, and bonks on the head that begin to negatively affect our spines. Even more importantly, it's our daily habits and routines that will have the greatest long-term impact.

▶ CHAPTER 2

HOW DO YOU GET BAD POSTURE?

When patients come to us in pain, they often want to know, "How did I get this way?" which they often follow with, "I didn't do anything. It just happened."

As we mentioned, there are only two ways to mess up your spine – trauma or a buildup of smaller traumas. The big traumas are more obvious – events like getting into a car accident or falling down some stairs. You would be surprised if you didn't get hurt when something like that happens.

We do tend to forget some of our many spinal traumas, especially when they occurred as kids. We're guessing you didn't learn how to walk on the first try, so there was a lot of wobbling and landing on your butt. If you did that now? Ouch.

What about learning to ride a bike? Did you do that correctly the first time, or were there some wobbles, falls, and crashes? If you fell off your bike now, you'd walk around for days with bruises, telling people all about that traumatic incident. As a kid, you likely did that on a regular basis and didn't think anything of it.

During our initial consultation, we ask patients about their history with sports. If they participated in any sports that involve collisions, there's a chance their spine suffered a trauma – at least enough trauma that one of their vertebrae could have moved out of place, become stuck, or both. Or perhaps they've spent years participating in a one-directional sport like golf, which will also take its toll over time.

On a smaller scale, maybe you like to sit a certain way that's not ideal but looks cool or is comfortable (*because your spine is already less than perfect, so it feels good*). The following are some anecdotes describing the interesting ways patients have caused their neck or back issues with smaller, seemingly insignificant, traumas:

- ⮑ A forty-year-old male patient comes to us with frequent low back pain that is worse on the right. He doesn't work at a computer, and he doesn't drive all day. His job requires that he walk a lot, but he's otherwise pretty balanced. After working through a list of possible issues, he tells us that his dog loves to play fetch and it's something they do every day. When the dog brings him back the ball, he bends down on his right knee to pick up the ball. Only his right knee. Every. Single. Time. This would be no big deal done only once, but doing it thirty to forty times a day, multiplied by several months was overdeveloping the muscles on one side of his body to the point that his pelvis kept twisting out of place. He kept his back pain from returning by kneeling with his left knee for a while and then later, alternating from side to side to keep things balanced.

- ⮑ One of our regular patients, a thirty-year-old female, had been doing great for months when she suddenly developed neck pain that was getting worse every day. After asking her about any new activities in her life, she remembered that she just moved to a new office. She had the same desk and chair as her prior office, so she didn't think anything of it at first. However, in the new office, there's an open door to her right, and every time someone walks past that door, she turns her head to look. She can't help it; she wants to know who is walking past the door. Over and over again she does this all day until she starts to build up the muscles on the right side of her neck, causing neck pain. Solution? She turned her desk so she could see straight out that door without turning her head.

- A male patient came in to see us with frequent low back pain. He does okay most of the day, but things get worse when he gets home and sits on the couch, watching TV with his girlfriend. After asking him about activities he does for extended periods, he realizes he always sits in the same spot on the couch. He sits at an angle so he can put his arm around his girlfriend and then turns his head to the right to watch TV. He did this for hours nearly every day until the back pain started. After some chiropractic care and showing him some exercises to counter what he's doing, he starts to feel better. He also moved to the other side of the couch. Problem solved.

- A female patient came in to see us with frequent headaches that had increased in frequency and intensity over the course of the past year. She had already been to several doctors and specialists, but no one was able to find anything wrong. Her daily activities include a lot of driving. We noticed she had her hair in a ponytail and asked her if she always wears her hair like that. She said she has for the past year or so because it finally got long enough. The ponytail was pushing her head forward while driving, causing a lot of extra strain and pressure at the back of her head. This daily strain – often for hours at a time – was leading to her recurring headaches. Chiropractic adjustments, exercises, and a new hairstyle did the trick. No more headaches.

- A forty-year-old male patient came to our office with occasional low back pain, but he felt a lot of pain in his hamstring. He'd been getting massages and doing physical therapy with no relief. An MRI examination showed there's nothing wrong with his hamstring, so he decided to see us. His X-rays showed that his spine was very twisted. During the examination, he asks how it got that way. Based on the X-rays, we show him what he must look like when he sits at his computer with his body one way and his screen to his right. His jaw drops open, and he says, "That's exactly how my desk is set up." That's why he developed back pain and hamstring pain – from twisting while sitting at the computer. Better ergonomics along with chiropractic care helped his problem.

These are just a few examples of the kinds of issues we deal with every day in our office. If your neck or back is hurting and you haven't experienced a major trauma, it's highly likely that your problem is coming from your everyday activities. It's time to play detective and figure out what you may be doing that's causing the imbalance and creating your problem.

> **BETTER POSTURE TIP:** See a chiropractor that takes X-rays and uses that information to evaluate your spine. While some people are hesitant to do this, hoping to avoid the X-rays and keep the costs down, you'd be amazed by how much information can be gathered from X-rays.

We tell patients, "If we followed you around all day, we would be able to figure out what you're doing that causes the problem because it's something you do repeatedly or something you do for extended periods." Today, patients usually (*but not always*) have decent ergonomics at their desks. They know to look for that. Big companies in our area hire ergonomic experts to make sure they are set up well at their desks, yet people still have bad posture because they do a lot of little things on a daily basis that can cause it. Very often, the activity that causes the problem is small and doesn't seem significant. Only when it's multiplied by weeks and months does it start to have an effect.

Sometimes it's just not possible for you to stop doing the imbalanced thing, like working at a computer. Even with perfect ergonomics, gravity is a constant force, and you'll still end up tightening and shortening the muscles in the front of your body more than the back. There's no other way to do your job, so what should you do? In cases like this, it's important that you work on stretches and exercises that counteract the effects of long hours at the computer.

We'll go into this in more detail, but essentially, you want to stretch tight areas and strengthen weak areas. Most patients just try to stretch everything because it feels good, but that won't solve the problem. And sometimes stretching areas that shouldn't be stretched actually makes the problem worse.

▶ CHAPTER 3

WHAT ARE THE EFFECTS OF BAD POSTURE?

We think we can say without exaggeration that bad posture is one of the leading causes of poor health. Yes, we're including neck and back pain, but there's a lot more to it. Your body is designed to work a specific way. You have two ears, two arms, and two legs, and they should all be level from side to side. In other words, your body should be balanced from side to side, and from front to back.

When your spine and body are in their best alignment, your body has its best chance to work and function in a healthy, pain-free way. Each degree of movement in the wrong direction may not cause pain or health problems, but it certainly increases the likelihood that the problems will eventually occur.

Depending on where you look and who you ask, bad posture can be the initial cause of any of the following health problems:

- Arthritis
- Back pain
- Carpal tunnel syndrome
- Chest pain
- Degenerative joint disease (DJD)
- Digestive problems
- Eye strain
- Herniated discs
- Hormone imbalances
- Fatigue
- Headaches
- Joint pain
- Muscle strain
- Neck pain
- Pain between the shoulder blades
- Repetitive stress injury (RSI)
- Respiratory problems
- Rotator cuff injury
- Sciatica
- Urinary/incontinence problems

To make matters worse, we can go our whole lives without realizing that any of the above problems are due to poor posture. You can take an aspirin for your headache or your back pain, see your doctor, get injections, or even have surgery and have no idea it all started with your bad posture.

Take a look at how drug companies spend their advertising dollars. Do they say anything about solving the cause of your problem? No. They strictly talk about your symptoms and the new anti-symptom chemical they have developed. If you cough, you get a cough suppressant without considering why your body needs to cough in the first place: the cough serves the purpose of clearing your throat. When we get a fever, we reach for acetaminophen or ibuprofen, but a fever destroys bacteria. We don't want to experience either a cough or a fever to a severe level, but maybe we shouldn't be so quick to stop our bodies from helping us out and telling us what's wrong.

Your doctor may run you through many treatments and tests to diagnose your condition, but they may never address how you got that way in the first place or what you can do to keep the problem from coming back. Addressing the cause will save you time, money, and poor health.

You could receive a lifetime of medications to cover up something that may be prevented by exercising ten minutes per day and changing some of your surroundings so you can perform your normal daily activities with more balanced movements.

Working on your posture is a great way to address the cause of your problem, rather than just the symptom. The unwanted conditions we listed above were caused by something. What caused it? How can you keep it from happening again? What if it's as simple as fixing your posture? How many symptoms can you help or prevent by improving your posture and your spine?

Let's take a look at the science behind one of the negative effects of the syndrome known as forward-head posture. It has been determined that an average head weighs approximately eight to ten pounds. (*Let's use ten pounds for this example.*) If your head is in its proper alignment over your shoulders, your spine acts like a big shock absorber, minimizing the strain and distributing the ten pounds of weight.

Gravity is always pulling on your head regardless of its position over your spine. However, with your head directly over your shoulders, the load on your spine is just the ten pounds. For every inch your head moves forward, the effective load on your spine increases by a factor of ten. A ten-pound head one inch in front of the shoulders is like having a twenty-pound head.

Move your head forward another inch, and your head will create thirty pounds of stress and strain on the muscles of your neck and back. After all, they are the muscles holding everything up, and they will bear the strain of the increase in weight.

Anyone that's ever pulled a baby out of a crib knows how much easier it is when the baby is close than when the baby is on the other side of the crib. The farther the baby is from you, the heavier they are to lift. Experiment with this at home using any item you can easily grip that's about ten pounds.

Hold it close and see how long you can hold it. You can probably hold it forever without getting tired. Now extend your arm and hold that same item at arm's length. How long can you hold it in this position? Thirty seconds? Why? The item didn't get heavier, but the way gravity pulled on it and the muscles being used to hold it changed dramatically.

How does this affect you long-term? When the load or pressure on your spine is increased, the bones will change to accommodate that increase. Typically, the bones will remodel by growing osteophytes, also known as bone spurs. Yikes! You definitely don't want to develop bone spurs if you can help it. Bone spurs are a permanent change to your spine and take years to develop.

The effects of bad posture don't begin in a subtle way, but they do develop in a way that can be covered up or ignored with common medications and methods. That thirty-pound head creates knots in your shoulder muscles. Then those two or three knots begin to make the entire neck and shoulder area tense and tight. Sound like anyone you know?

Meanwhile, the bones underneath are slowly and steadily creating the bone spurs that will shut down the joint that's not functioning correctly or that's no longer able to support your activities with just the muscles.

Your body gives you warning signs, which we tend to tune out. Please, don't do that. Recognize what your body is trying to tell you and use that information to make a change for the better.

Some studies indicate that some posture syndromes can alter the amount of blood flow to the spinal cord. Some positions have been known to cause disc damage. Poor postural mechanics can affect your rib cage, stopping your ability to take in all the oxygen you might need each time you inhale.

That's a lot of stuff that can happen with bad posture, wouldn't you agree? Later we'll talk about some of the devastating effects of bad posture. These are the types of conditions we see in our office every day.

> **BETTER POSTURE TIP:** When dealing with posture or health issues, look to the cause of the problem when seeking a solution, don't just focus on the symptoms. Covering up a symptom with medications isn't a good long-term strategy.

> CHAPTER 4

DIAGNOSE YOUR POSTURE PROBLEM

Now it's time to take a hard look at your posture. It's not enough to determine that you have bad posture; you need to figure out what exactly is bad about it so that you can fix it and measure your results.

The first step is a postural analysis. What do you think needs your attention? This is a difficult process to get totally straight on your own, so we suggest you find someone to help you take a look. Alternatively, you can take a photo standing as normally as you can, trying to capture your entire body in the shot.

Get a head start on the analysis by looking at yourself in the mirror. Do your

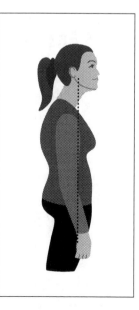

shoulders seem to roll forward, or are they back? Can you even move them back if you want to, or are they stuck?

Compare the level of your ears side to side. Check the height of each shoulder. Are they even side to side? Lastly, dig into your sides – the "love handle" areas – and feel for the tops of your pelvis. Once you've found them on each side, mark the top with your hands. Now you have a rough idea about the height of your pelvis from side to side.

These three body parts (*ears, shoulders, pelvis*) are good posture landmarks to use to evaluate how you're doing from the front. Are you wondering how you're going to check yourself from the side on your own? Other than rigging up some sort of camera/mirror combo, it's easiest to find a helper.

Stand as naturally as possible (*you can try again to attempt your best possible posture*), and take a look. Your most natural posture is obviously more likely to represent how you look most of the time during your normal activities.

Your earlobe should line up with your shoulder, which should line up with your hip down to your ankle. Does your posture do that?

FORWARD HEAD POSTURE

If your earlobe is in front of your shoulders, you likely have forward-head posture, though it's possible that your earlobe will still line up with your shoulders if your shoulders are rolled forward. You can use your hips or ankles as another point of reference in this case.

Do you see evidence that you have this posture syndrome? If so, then you will benefit from neck exercises (*don't worry, we will share what the right exercises later in this book*). Once the neck muscles become strained, leaning your head over for even short periods of time can lead to neck pain.

People develop forward head posture most often from looking down at their phones or having their computer monitors too low.

Your head is heavy! Over time your neck muscles get tighter in the front and longer in the back.

Changing this bad posture position means lengthening the muscles in the front of your neck and strengthening the muscles in the back of your neck. But what do most people do? They never exercise to strengthen the relevant muscles, and they pull down on the back of their head to stretch the back of their neck, which will only make their forward-head posture worse. The crazy part is, the stretching makes them feel good temporarily, so they just keep doing it.

Proper posture enables strained neck and back muscles to heal more quickly, and forward-head posture is fixable unless the spine has already started to make permanent degenerative changes. Take action sooner, rather than later if you want to stop this posture problem in its tracks.

ROUNDED SHOULDERS

Are your shoulders in front of your head, hip, and ankle? Are you having trouble rolling your shoulders back? Are you already beginning to show signs of hyperkyphosis (*i.e., the "hump"*)?

If your shoulders are rounded, you need to stretch the chest muscles and strengthen your upper back muscles. Rounded shoulders usually result from slouching and keeping your arms in front of you (*which you have to do all day when using a computer*).

When slouching, the natural forward curve of the neck is exaggerated, which often results in neck pain and upper back pain. Slouching is more common when sitting, and it's often caused by fatigue, especially when sitting in front of a computer.

Rounding your shoulders will also lead to limitations in thoracic mobility. That means you won't have normal movement in your upper and mid-back. This can lead to overuse of and limitations in your shoulders that can lead to injuries.

Thoracic mobility can also be improved with chiropractic adjustments, a foam roller, and other mobility options. Don't worry, we'll cover all of that soon.

THE "HUMP"

Particularly with osteoporosis, vertebrae become fragile and fracture. If the fracture occurs in the front half of the vertebra (*more common with typical bad postural positions and the increased stress with that posture*), the vertebra above will begin to tilt forward.

This tilt continues to increase the likelihood of additional fractures, more tilting, and further advancement of the "Dowager's hump." If you're developing the hump, you need to go after this condition from all fronts: nutritionally, with chiropractic care, with exercise, and with posture supports.

Some patients will start to see fatty deposits occurring on the upper back, making the hump even more pronounced. These deposits can go away with weight loss, but they will become increasingly less obvious as your posture improves.

The dowager's hump is painful and can be a permanent condition. If you even think you're likely to get one, or if you're already showing signs of developing one, it's time to take action!

SWAYBACK

Hyperlordosis, also known as "swayback," is the name given to the posture condition of having too much curve in your lower back. This can be accentuated in someone who has more belly fat, but it can occur in anyone.

While swayback may be indicative of a spinal condition called spondylolisthesis (*covered in this book*), you can address this posture problem with chiropractic care, stretches, and exercises.

These conditions we've just described in this section are the primary posture conditions we see in our office, and they can all be improved in a short period of time. You can have Better Posture Fast and change all of these conditions with the right plan of attack.

CHAPTER 5

CONDITIONS THAT CAN LEAD TO & BE CAUSED BY BAD POSTURE

DEGENERATIVE JOINT DISEASE

Because we're chiropractors, degenerative joint disease in the spine is an area of particular interest to us and one of the most common conditions we see in our office. It's concerning how quickly patients will dismiss seeing degeneration on their X-rays: "Oh, that's common for someone my age, right?"

It may be "common," but that doesn't make it "normal" or even "ideal." Spinal

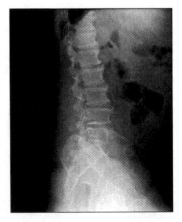

degeneration does not just form when you turn a certain age. "Age of the problem" is a more accurate way of seeing the severity in spinal degeneration, not "age of the person." You don't have to have degenerative joint disease.

It is common for us to see an area of spinal degeneration at the same spinal level where the patient is having their pain. A patient will tell me, "I have pain right here," and I often end up showing them an X-ray that has degeneration at that same spinal level. The symptoms may have just shown up, but the problem has clearly been there longer. The degeneration is the evidence of the age of the problem.

The interesting thing about this is that degenerative joint disease (*DJD*) is not a painful process when it begins. You can go from having a totally normal spine to a spine that is degenerating, to one where the bones have fused – and you may never have felt any symptoms at all! Let's say that again. You can have a vertebra with a problem, have bone spurs form, and have your spinal joints fuse beyond repair without ever experiencing pain or a symptom of any kind.

Degenerative joint disease is evidence of a long-term spinal problem, but it doesn't cause pain all by itself. DJD does not form overnight; it takes years. Effectively, your spine has to function poorly and continue to function poorly for a long time in order for DJD to become bad enough to be evident on your X-rays.

We believe our patients when they tell us, "My pain just started last week," but that doesn't change the fact that while the symptoms started last week, the problem began a long time ago. Changes that are visible on an X-ray don't show up that quickly.

It is entirely possible that those people sitting in front of a computer all day will one day wake up with pain so bad they have to seek professional help, only to find that they have a spine filled with bone spurs and degeneration. They will believe that the problem only just started, when in fact it's only the pain that just started.

DJD is known as "wear and tear" arthritis, so consider this analogy of driving around with your wheels out of alignment: The evidence of the misalignment shows up in your tires, not your wheels, and it can take a while. You can look for uneven tire wear as proof that your wheels are out of alignment. You can replace your tires in an attempt to fix the problem, but your tires will just wear out quickly again until you address the wheel alignment. You can't replace your spine, which means you have to get it back into alignment. (*That's what chiropractors do.*)

In addition, DJD results not only from the misalignment of your spine, but also from bad posture and the lack of good function. You don't always feel or see the poor function; you just eventually see the evidence on an X-ray. Symptoms of DJD don't always have to be pain, although that's a very motivating one.

Consider this: We had an elderly patient come back to see us after a five-year absence. She could barely speak; she sounded like she was whispering. She had been like that for months and had already been to several doctors and had a bunch of tests performed, including an endoscopy. She's in her late sixties, but very active and in great health. They couldn't find anything wrong other than "normal" spinal degeneration in her middle back.

As a "What could it hurt?" option, she decided to see if it was something related to her spine. She told us, "I figured even if my voice didn't come back, at least my back would feel better." She had some restrictions in the movement of her spine, particularly in the mid-back area. She was adjusted, and for about a day, her voice came back. She returned a few days later, whispering again. She was adjusted over the next few weeks, and her voice has been back for several years now without issue. We share this story because it was the dysfunction of her spine that caused a symptom unrelated to pain.

If her back hurt, she would have thought about coming back to see us and would have known we could help, but she didn't make the connection to her spine for this particular symptom. Of course, we had the benefit of all the other tests she had had and doctors she had seen. We knew there wasn't anything going on inside her that needed help beyond what we could do in our office.

The process of DJD starts with an area of the spine becoming stuck and not functioning properly, and then advances to wearing out the joint's surface. This is followed by bone spurs, narrowing of the joint space, hardening of the bone at the joint surface, and deformity of the joint.

DJD is also known as osteoarthritis, OA, and osteoarthrosis. If you do get symptoms, they may include joint stiffness, pain, and limitation in the joint's normal ranges of motion (like when your neck turns great to the left, but not so well to the right). However, if your body is "just not working right," that's a good enough reason to get checked out.

HERNIATED DISCS

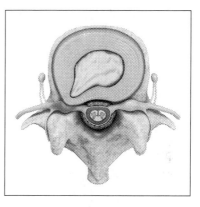

Another potentially negative effect of bad posture is a herniated disc (*sometimes referred to as a "slipped" disc or a "ruptured" disc*). Your spinal discs are rubbery pads found between your vertebrae. The inner portion of the disc is filled with a jelly-like substance, while the outer ring is more cartilage-like. The discs act as shock absorbers for your spine.

When the spine is in its best alignment, the amount of stress on the disc is evenly distributed across the entire disc. When the spine moves out of alignment, increased stress and pressure are placed on some portions of the disc. Since the disc is filled with a jelly-like substance, as you increase pressure on one side of it, the jelly eventually has to go somewhere. A disc is said to have herniated when the center jelly pushes through the outer edge of the disc. This can create pressure in the center, affecting the spinal cord, or it can create pressure to the side on spinal nerves. Because spinal nerves are very sensitive to pressure, the pressure inevitably leads to pain, numbness, tingling, or weakness.

If you spend too much time in a hunched-over position (*e.g., in a bad postural position*), eventually something has to give – the jelly-like substance between your vertebrae starts to push out, creating pressure on a nerve. If you have a disc bulging out to the side, you are likely leaning off to one side to take pressure off it. You may not even realize you're doing it at first, but the longer you sit, stand, and do activities with irregular posture to avoid pain, the worse it gets.

Patients experiencing pain from bulging or herniated discs are very common in our office, and this is a condition we love to treat. Helping patients with this problem can help them avoid taking medications long-term or even surgery. Helping patients feel better is one thing, but helping patients avoid surgery is a great reason to be a chiropractor.

In addition to bad posture, other activities can weaken the disc. Still, most of the following activities create extra pressure on the disc because the person is performing the activity with improper posture.

The activities include:

- Improper lifting or lifting something awkwardly
- Excessive body weight
- Physical trauma
- Twisting with weight
- Sitting for extended periods

Symptoms of a herniated disc include:

- Pain
- Weakness in one extremity (*arm or leg*)
- Numbness or tingling ("*pins and needles*") in one extremity
- Loss of bowel or bladder control (*this is considered an emergency situation – get to a hospital!*)
- Burning pain
- Increased pain with flexed movements, like bending forward or looking down

- ➲ Increased pain when bearing down, like when using the restroom
- ➲ Increased pain when coughing, laughing, or sneezing

Not all neck and back pain is the result of a herniated disc. Numbness and tingling can be caused by many other conditions. Irritation, inflammation, or swelling in the disc can cause many of the same symptoms as a herniated disc. Swelling in the disc may be a precursor to a herniated disc and may cause nearly all the same symptoms.

You cannot diagnose a herniated disc on your own. Your health professional will likely begin with a physical examination followed by X-rays and/or an MRI examination to arrive at the best diagnosis. While the doctor will be able to tell whether the disc is involved without advanced diagnostic tests, the tests will pinpoint exactly where the disc is herniated and how severe the condition is.

The term "herniated disc" is super-scary to most of our patients. Once they hear it, they begin to worry and run off as quickly as possible to a surgeon. However, there are alternatives to caring for a herniated disc that do not involve surgery (*including chiropractic adjustments, physical therapy, spinal decompression, and steroid injections*). Sometimes, though, surgery is required.

We find we can help 80-90 percent of our disc patients avoid more invasive treatment. Some will get some kind of injection as a next step if they're not seeing results with chiropractic care, while only a small percentage are referred for surgery. In nearly every surgical case we've seen, the patient simply waited too long before seeking help other than medications.

Medications

Some patients are prescribed medications to control pain or to decrease inflammation, and sometimes muscle relaxers are prescribed. Keep in mind that covering up symptoms with medications can lead to further problems. How can a pill put your spine back in place? How can a medication improve your posture? Pills just can't do that.

When taking medications for neck or back pain, the best result you can hope for is that the decrease in inflammation will give your disc a chance to heal. Also, managing the pain can give you a chance to do something about some of the structural problems that may be contributing to the condition.

Chiropractic and Physical Therapy

Depending on the severity of the herniated disc, chiropractic and physical therapy should be considered prior to ever seriously considering surgery. In most cases, your medical doctor will recommend physical therapy, not chiropractic care. We find that this is a mistake.

A combination of chiropractic care and physical therapy work very well together. Physical therapy may include stretches and exercises, as well as home-care exercises and recommendations. A physical therapist may also include treatments such as electrical stimulation, ice, heat, and ultrasound, which many chiropractors can also provide.

If you are referred for physical therapy and aren't seeing results but still want to explore every option before surgery, then you should strongly consider chiropractic. Some patients are afraid to visit a chiropractor, but they will readily take medications that have known side effects or undergo surgery with its risks and complications.

There are many ways to adjust the spine, so don't run to surgery without exploring all your options first. If you're worried about "pops" and "cracks," just ask your chiropractor to use a different technique. There are many ways to adjust the spine, and some are gentler than others. The gentle versions may not yield a satisfying "crack," but they can still get great results.

Spinal Decompression Therapy

Although many health insurance companies still consider spinal decompression therapy experimental or investigational, we see great results with our patients using it. There are many types of spinal decompression devices, but the general idea is the machine specifically pulls on the vertebrae on either side of the affected disc.

This pulling, subsequent releasing, then pulling again creates a vacuum effect that allows the jelly-like disc material to return to the proper area of the disc. It's not uncommon for patients to feel near immediate relief when the machine pulls them out the first time. You have to start gently, but the machines can pull stronger and stronger on subsequent visits, if needed.

This therapy is not covered by health insurance and prices can vary widely among providers offering this service. You should receive an X-ray before using this device, as different spinal conditions need to be decompressed in different ways. Expect to do a series of visits to get better results.

Injections

Epidural steroid injections are another common stepping-stone in the process of treating and resolving herniated discs. Usually, the injections are performed in a series of three, with the medication being injected directly into the area of herniation.

Injections require an MRI examination first so that the doctor can see exactly where the disc is herniated. The procedure may be done at a surgical or diagnostic center because the doctor will require fluoroscopy to help guide the needle into the right place. You do not want the doctor making their best guess when administering this injection. It needs to be very specific.

Some research reports that receiving this type of injection may prevent the disc from fully healing, as it can block some of the body's natural healing factors that will help the disc recover. However, if you're in a ton of pain, can't find a comfortable position, your medications aren't doing the trick, and/or you want to avoid surgery – this is still an option.

We would still recommend that you keep trying to address the cause of the problem, taking advantage of any pain relief provided by the injections to improve your spinal alignment and strengthen the supporting muscles. Once the injection wears off (*in months or years*), patients may find themselves feeling worse than before if they've just gone back to doing bad stuff for their spine and not fixing the issue.

Surgery

Spinal surgeries should be your absolute last option. Unfortunately, we see many patients undergo surgery because their insurance will pay for it, and they avoid alternatives because they aren't covered. While price is certainly a factor, the risk of long-term problems with spinal surgeries should be a real concern.

There are times when we have to tell a patient that they must see a surgeon for a consultation. Most often this is because the damage to the disc has progressed too far and damaged the nerve. A common symptom of this type of damage is weakness down their arm or leg. In these cases, avoiding the surgery could lead to a permanent change in their nerve. You have to get the pressure off the nerve to avoid permanent damage, so surgery cannot be avoided in every case.

Thankfully, we find we need to refer only one or two cases a year for surgery, and we are able to handle many cases conservatively. We do work with medical doctors that are also conservative and who do not look to surgery as the first option. Having a good group of doctors that try to address herniated discs without surgery will save you from any unnecessary and risky procedures.

> **BETTER POSTURE TIP:** Sometimes surgery is necessary, but it shouldn't be your first option. You can always get surgery for a back problem. However, once you have surgery, you've often eliminated many of your conservative options. Chiropractic first, drugs second, and surgery last.

LEG-LENGTH DEFICIENCY

"Doc, it feels like one of my legs is longer than the other."

In chiropractic school, we were taught that leg-length differences were more likely to be a functional difference than an anatomical one. This means that if your pelvis shifts out of place, it can pull the femur (*hip joint*) up with it and make one side seem shorter as a result, which is something we see all day, every day. If your pelvis twists one way, the spine will deviate to create balance for the rest of your body, thus causing bad posture. This is a functional difference, as it doesn't mean your legs are different lengths.

The problem is, what if the difference in your leg length is not due to a misalignment of the pelvis? What if it's actually shorter?

Traditional methods will have the health care provider (*usually a chiropractor or physical therapist*) determine the leg-length discrepancy by measuring each leg with a tape measure and comparing the distances. This is not a very accurate or reliable way to go about it, in our experience. We're looking for millimeters of difference, so it's important to be as accurate as possible.

We take a special X-ray in our office that captures the hip joint, knee joint, and ankle joint all in one shot. The X-ray is taken with a ruler behind it, which we use as a reference point. We measure the upper leg (*femur*) and the lower leg (*tibia*) to get accurate measurements, then we take the measurement of one leg and subtract it from the measurement of the other leg. Just like that, we can see the discrepancy between your legs down to the millimeter.

If the difference between your legs is less than 3 mm, we won't typically add anything to the inside of your shoe. If the difference is between 3 and 5 mm (*the most common difference we see*), then we will add a heel lift to the inside of your shoe to even things out.

If the difference between your legs is more than 5 mm, you have some choices to make. We can add heel lifts of 7-9 mm or a full-length shoe insert that goes up to 18 mm, but they won't fit in all shoes. You may find that you need to increase your shoe size or not choose low-rise shoes to allow for the additional insert.

Some patients just add the most they can without changing their shoes entirely, and they still feel much better than they did before adding the insert. If the difference is big enough, it's a good choice to consider having your shoes modified on the outside to make up the difference.

These big differences are rare and don't always cause pain. If you find that your neck and back pain just won't go away or your posture changes don't seem to last, or if you just feel like your legs are different lengths, this may be the cause.

We began to treat patients for this condition when we noticed some patients seemed to have the same misalignment over and over again. It would stand to reason that if we performed a chiropractic adjustment to the same spot and in the same direction over and over again, it should eventually stay. When it didn't, we continued to investigate anatomical leg length discrepancies.

While not all patients have this issue, many patients have a difference that will require at least a small heel lift to help them stay in the right posture.

> **BETTER POSTURE TIP:** If it feels like your legs are different lengths, they probably are. You'll need to get evaluated to find out if that discrepancy is functional (*can be adjusted out*) or anatomical (*will need a special insert or shoe*). Resolving this issue can make all the difference when it comes to avoiding both long-term spinal changes and neck and back pain.

ROTATOR CUFF INJURIES

Your "rotator cuff" refers to the muscles and tendons of your shoulder joint that make it move. There are four major muscles that make up the "cuff": the subscapularis, the supraspinatus, the infraspinatus, and the teres minor. (*Don't worry, there won't be a quiz.*)

The tendons of these muscles connect to your humerus (*the bone of your upper arm*) and your scapula (*shoulder blade*). They help move and rotate your shoulder, but they also help to hold it in place and provide stability.

Your shoulder is the most mobile joint in your entire body, capable of moving in nearly every direction. This increased mobility, however, causes a decrease in stability. This means that if you are using your shoulder to make only a couple of its movements all the time, the other muscles can become weak, which destabilizes the shoulder even more.

Can you really hurt your shoulder with bad posture? Absolutely. We have had patients with non-active lifestyles come in with rotator cuff tears who have experienced no known trauma. That is, they couldn't remember or describe any time in which they "pulled" their shoulder or fell down or anything like that.

Instead, the trauma was their bad posture. Of their four rotator cuff muscles, one (*usually the supraspinatus*) was not getting the strengthening it needed, while it was being stretched and strained repeatedly by shoulders that were rolling forward.

Gravity kept pulling and pulling on the shoulder joint until something finally had to give. That "give" occurred in the form of a tear, and pain was the result.

More commonly, rotator cuff injuries are the result of falling, lifting, and/or repetitive arm movement (*especially overhead movements*). In other words, having bad posture for years is the equivalent of suffering a bad fall. Interesting.

Signs and symptoms that you may have a rotator cuff injury include the following:

- ⮑ Pain and tenderness in your shoulder joint
- ⮑ Painful shoulder movements, especially reaching overhead, reaching behind your back, lifting and pulling

- Pain when you sleep on that shoulder
- Shoulder weakness
- Decrease in your shoulder's range of motion
- The tendency to avoid doing things with your shoulder

You may not even recognize that you have limited ranges of motion in your shoulder. Take this simple test: Can you scratch all areas of your own back? Are there large sections that you simply can't reach?

How about putting on your bra? Are you able to put on your bra with the hooks in the back? We hear from our patients on a regular basis that they don't have enough mobility in their shoulders to fasten their bra with the hooks in the back, so they have to put their bra on with the hooks in the front. They have gotten so used to doing this that they don't realize how limited their shoulder range of motion has become.

Treatment for this injury includes therapy, steroid injections, and surgery. Most rotator cuff injuries are treated with physical therapy to strengthen the specific muscles that are weak and with certain modalities that decrease inflammation and speed up healing.

Essentially, the treatment is to provide more balance to your shoulder joint that was undone with your bad posture. This is something you can help prevent now by improving the overall strength and stability of your rotator cuff.

We work with patients on shoulder mobility and range of motion on a regular basis. There are chiropractic adjustments that specifically address the primary bones of the shoulder (*humerus, clavicle, scapula*) and their joints.

You'd be surprised how much range of motion you can get back with some adjustments to those areas. However, if the muscles of the rotator cuff are torn, you'll need to address the tear. Repairing a minor tear may involve just rest and ice. Major tears may require surgery if they can't be resolved conservatively.

FROZEN SHOULDER

We've been seeing more frozen shoulders lately, and the origin of this problem appears to be directly related to bad posture. When you hunch over, your shoulders tend to roll forward. Trying to do your normal daily activities with your shoulders rolling forward causes pain and injury.

If it hurts to reach overhead, guess what you'll avoid doing. You will avoid reaching overhead at first because it hurts, but not using your shoulder's full range of motion eventually leads to restrictions that prevent you from doing that movement at all. It truly is a "use it or lose it" scenario when it comes to your range of motion.

Over time, your shoulder muscles will develop adhesions, preventing your shoulder from moving even further. We have patients that haven't lifted their arm above eye level in years. They finally come to see us when they can barely lift it over their belly button.

Chiropractors can help a lot with shoulder movement, but there can come a point when frozen shoulder syndrome requires more invasive treatment. A common treatment involves manipulation under anesthesia. You are put under anesthesia, and then the doctor moves your shoulder joint around to break up the adhesions. The procedure is far too painful to do without the anesthesia.

Frozen shoulder syndrome is gradually acquired, and it can be a lot of work to undo once you have it. The key here is to not ignore your limited range of motion, but to work to improve it.

An easy test is to stand in front of a wall holding a small piece of tape in the hand of your bad shoulder. Raise your arm as high as you can, and put the tape at that level. Once a week, make sure you can go at least that high again with your arm. Of course, it's much better if you can go higher, but you want to make sure that you're at least not losing ground.

If you find that you can't reach that level, it's time to really get after your frozen shoulder before it requires invasive methods to help "unfreeze" it.

One of our patients with a frozen shoulder only noticed it while playing golf. He just couldn't get the right range of motion. During his regular daily activities of working at the computer, he couldn't even tell he had a problem. That's the insidious nature of losing range of motion. If you don't use your body in different ways, you may not even notice that you can't do certain things. Improving posture and working on balanced activities can save you a lot of pain and problems.

Like spinal joints, the joints of the shoulder can also be adjusted. Not all chiropractors feel comfortable adjusting beyond the spine, but most do. The chiropractor will address all three bones of the shoulder and their joints to make sure they are moving well. If they're not, a simple adjustment can make an almost immediate improvement in the shoulder's range of motion.

> **BETTER POSTURE TIP:** Get shoulder problems addressed early, especially if you notice you have limited range of motion. The longer you wait, the more likely you are to develop a frozen shoulder. Stretches, exercises, mobility work, and chiropractic adjustments can make a big difference.

SCOLIOSIS

First of all, we want to emphasize that spinal misalignments and scoliosis are not the same thing. Many patients come to our office concerned that they have scoliosis. When we take an X-ray that reveals that their curves are not as they should be, their first assumption is that they have scoliosis. Anything more than a ten-degree curve is considered scoliosis, but it doesn't mean you will become disfigured or will need invasive interventions.

Scoliosis is largely hereditary. If someone in your family has scoliosis, it's not a guarantee that that you'll get it too, but it certainly increases the chances (*by about 20 percent*). The vast majority of scoliosis cases are called "idiopathic," which is a fancy way of saying "unknown cause." Idiopathic scoliosis usually develops prior to puberty and is more prevalent in girls than boys.

Scoliosis can develop in adults, but it is usually a non-diagnosed and/or non-treated version of a childhood condition. Adult scoliosis can also develop as a result of spinal deformities and complications resulting from osteoporosis, namely compression fractures of the vertebrae.

Parents should watch for the following signs of scoliosis in their children, but it's possible you have some of these indicators as well. Not everyone has had their scoliosis detected or treated. (*if you think you have any of these, you may also question whether you just have bad posture or bad posture with scoliosis*):

- ⮑ Uneven shoulders
- ⮑ Uneven base of the head (*sometimes your earrings make this more noticeable*)
- ⮑ Prominent shoulder blade or shoulder blades (*this is a very common symptom*)
- ⮑ Uneven or twisted waistline
- ⮑ Your nose and belly button don't line up
- ⮑ Elevated hips
- ⮑ Leaning to one side

If a scoliotic curve is severe when it is first seen, or if treatment with a brace does not control the curve, surgery may be necessary. There are scoliosis-focused chiropractors out there who have treated this condition with great success. As always, surgery should be considered only as a last option – please!

While surgery is sometimes necessary, we're shocked by how quickly people are willing to put screws, plates, and bolts in their spine. These surgeries are no small procedure, have risks, include long-term side effects, and shouldn't be considered as the first option.

DOWAGER'S HUMP

While a significant trauma can absolutely cause a spinal fracture, a spinal fracture due to a complication from osteoporosis causes a dowager's hump. Essentially, the bone becomes weak and then begins to collapse under your body weight. This most commonly occurs in the upper and mid-back. The fractured vertebra compresses more at the front of the bone, causing the upper back to curve more; thus, it forms "the hump."

Often the fracture is never diagnosed and is only found years later on an X-ray. The main symptom of a spinal fracture is back pain, usually in the upper or mid-back. Because the back pain is similar to any other strain or common back injury, the patient takes their medications and hopes the pain goes away ... and it does.

Fractures – even a spinal fracture – heal like anything else. However, a spinal fracture heals compressed, no longer shaped as it was. The patient continues to have weak bones, and they have one less vertebra to support their weight, which leads to more spinal fractures as the patient, leaning forward, puts even more strain on their spine.

Spinal fractures caused by osteoporosis often occur while doing an activity that causes relatively minor trauma to the spine, such as an insignificant fall, or twisting while lifting. Even such activities as sneezing, coughing, or turning over in bed can lead to compression or rib fractures in patients with advanced osteoporosis.

Ultimately, it's these fractures that severely alter the shape of the spine, leading to thoracic hyperkyphosis, also known as a dowager's hump. Avoiding osteoporosis is obviously a key component to decreasing your chance of spinal fracture.

Before you get osteoporosis, you should think of it like putting bone density into a bank. At some point in your life, you will definitely lose more bone strength than you gain. The more you have in the "bank," the less it will affect you.

Eating healthy, lifting weights, doing weight-bearing exercises, not smoking, and avoiding soda will all help you keep as much bone strength as possible. Thankfully, more women are consistently lifting weights than ever before, getting stronger in their bones, ligaments, tendons, joints, and muscles. This will help a lot in avoiding the dowager's hump.

Improving your posture and decreasing the strain on weak vertebrae are also extremely important when it comes to avoiding this problem. It's one thing to make the bones stronger; it's another to stop creating so much strain on them during your day. Hunching over, looking down at your phone, and slouching all put increased pressure on your spinal joints.

A common way that dowager's hump patients keep their spine from collapsing further is with the use of a posture or support brace for their upper back. We'll talk more later about the negative effects of using a brace long-term, but in this case, it's the right choice.

As an additional support for patients with osteoporosis, braces are key to avoiding further compression fractures in the spine. The best treatment is to not have to do treatment at all by avoiding this problem altogether. The next best choice is to support the spine, decrease the strain on it, and then work on strengthening it as much as you can.

The exercises and stretches we describe later in the book can be helpful in reversing the effects of the dowager's hump, decreasing pain, and improving posture.

> **BETTER POSTURE TIP:** Taking action to avoid osteoporosis should happen as early in life as possible. We highly recommend weight-bearing exercises and lifting weights to increase the density of your bones. Talk with your doctor and a trainer before starting any exercise program.

MISSHAPEN VERTEBRAE

Although this condition doesn't manifest in a lot of people, there are some who were born with a vertebra or vertebrae that are shaped abnormally. While this may not be life-threatening, painful, or even noticeable, it may cause poor posture. (*If you know you have misshapen vertebrae, and if you also have bad posture, that doesn't mean that that particular vertebra is the cause of your posture problems.*)

However, if you are working to improve your posture and your efforts just don't seem to be making any difference, you may be working with a structural problem that cannot be exercised back into place.

Let's not totally disregard the right exercises for you just because you think that maybe, possibly, you have a misshapen vertebra. You'll need to visit your family doctor or chiropractor to get an X-ray to be sure. (*This is yet another reason why we take x-rays before adjusting our patients in most cases.*)

We still believe that even if the bones of your spine are not symmetrical and are giving you the tendency to lean one way or another, you can do a lot with the right exercises and stretches to reduce the strain on your spine and stay as even, neutral, and straight as you can. In addition, maintaining a lean body mass is also helpful so that there is not any excessive weight to exaggerate imbalances on a spine that is misshapen.

SPONDYLOLISTHESIS

Spondylolisthesis is a condition of the spine in which one vertebra "slips" over the vertebra below it. There are various causes behind this condition, including a stress fracture to a part of the vertebra and age-related degenerative changes. Most practitioners believe, however, that this condition requires a trauma of some kind, even if it happened in childhood. Most patients that have spondylolisthesis know they had something bad happen at that spot in their spine.

A stress fracture in a vertebra may cause it to disconnect from its facet joints. The vertebra slips forward, leading to misalignment and narrowing of the spinal canal. Because this condition cannot typically be detected with a regular physical examination, an X-ray is needed to indicate the level involved and the severity.

From a posture standpoint, patients will report they feel pain when they put their head back or lean back with their lower spine. You may feel like your lower back is hyperlordotic (*has too much curve*), sometimes referred to as a swayback.

Spondylolisthesis usually responds well to conservative treatment, including chiropractic care and spinal decompression. Surgery is rarely needed unless you continue to do activities that can potentially increase how much the vertebra is slipping.

If you have had recurring low back pain and have never had an X-ray, this is another great reason to have one. Your doctor can't tell by looking at you if you have a spondylolisthesis, but an X-ray will let them know right away.

BETTER POSTURE TIP: If you are experiencing back pain (particularly sharp pain) following exercises where your spine goes into extension (leaning back), spondylolisthesis should be considered as a complicating factor as to why your neck and back pain doesn't seem to go away. Consult with your chiropractor or medical doctor to find out if you have one.

▶ CHAPTER 6

HOW TO DO EVERYDAY ACTIVITIES WITH GOOD POSTURE

Bad posture starts out as a bad habit, something you begin doing as a result of your normal daily activities. After all, we can't imagine anyone wishing that their shoulders would roll forward or their head would jut out. Your posture problem may have started with a lack of confidence – you just started hanging your head down.

We see teenagers slumping just because they're teenagers or because they're looking down at their phones. They spend hours with their laptop in their laps, sitting on the couch. We see tall kids slouching to appear more similar in height to their peers and teenage girls folding their arms and slouching forward to hide their growing chests.

Whether it was due to a lack of confidence or a way to fit in, this may be what started you down the path to bad posture.

If you happen to survive with good posture into your adult years, your chosen job or occupation may begin to wear you down. Take a look at your typical daily activities. You do almost the same things every single day. You may be working on different projects, but you still just sit in front of the computer all day, or at least in the same position all day.

Maybe your workstation is set up for a person who's five feet tall, but you're five-foot-ten and are straining to fit into your confined surroundings. Your chair may be top-of-the-line, but not suitable for someone with your back condition or routine.

Maybe your normal daily activities include going home and plopping down into a comfortable but non-supportive couch every night and holding that position until your four to six hours of favorite shows run their course.

Here's another way to think about it: Let's say you go to the gym and only do dumbbell curls to build up your biceps. That's it. Day after day, week after week, you only work on your biceps. Would your biceps build up? Sure they would!

The opposing muscle that creates balance in your upper arm is the triceps. Would your triceps build up? Of course not. You may get some residual benefits from lifting or carrying the weight around, but you will be creating a very unbalanced upper arm.

It's only a matter of time before your biceps become stronger and shorter while your triceps become longer and weaker. Eventually something's going to give.

To avoid this problem, all you have to do is work the opposing muscle to counteract the muscle that is being worked all the time. How much more? That depends on the results you get. It's entirely possible that you need to work your triceps twice as often (*or more!*) as your biceps to get good results. You have to watch and look for balance.

Posture is no different. If you are driving to work each day, sitting at a computer all day, then driving home and sitting on the couch, all your activities are being done in front of you. There is virtually no opportunity for your back muscles to work or grow stronger.

What's going to happen? Your front muscles will become shorter and stronger while your back muscles become longer and weaker … and the path to bad posture begins.

Bad posture is the result of the muscles tugging and pulling on your spine. If you work lots of muscles in the front of your body and not the back, you will have a hunched-over body. If you strengthen your back muscles and not your front, you will end up bent over backwards! (*This will never happen because you do almost every activity in front of you. The muscles in the front of your body will always be used more frequently during your day than the muscles in your back.*)

To support the human skeleton, our bodies are designed with quick-fire muscles that are meant to contract, sustaining muscles that are more supportive, and ligaments that allow for some movement but maintain the closeness of the bones.

The activities you do during the day determine the strength, flexibility, and balance of your spine. If you have lots of diversity in your daily movements and you sit, stand, and workout frequently and intensely for good posture, you probably have great posture.

If you sit or stand for long periods and don't work out, then you probably have that hunched-over posture. It would make sense that if you spend most of your day bent forward and you add in exercises that strengthen the front of your body, you will end up with an even more hunched-over posture.

Simply making changes to your normal routine that provide some variety and give your back muscles a chance to catch up will make a huge difference in how you look and feel.

Strengthen the muscles that support your back from all angles. Bring balance to your body by finding your weak areas and strengthening them. Find tight and restricted areas and spend time loosening the tight areas and lengthening the restricted or shortened muscles.

It is important to have enough strength to sustain your posture all day long. The goal isn't to make everyone into a bodybuilder, but to make the muscles strong enough to hold up your head and keep your shoulders back.

Perfect posture is within your reach if you take the time to counteract what you can't stop doing – the stuff you have to do every day. In no way should you stop doing the things that you need to do to get through your day. Taking notice of how you do those things and keeping things balanced will go a long, long way to improving your posture.

The good news is that it doesn't take eight hours of exercise to counteract eight hours of bad posture. Positive results can happen with some changes to your habits and the addition of just a few minutes of exercise daily.

The following are some general tips to help you improve your posture and to use good ergonomics to reduce the strain on your spinal joints.

Know the Warning Signs

Back pain is often the first symptom that your spine is being affected by poor posture or poor ergonomics. Back pain that is worse after a long day of sitting in your office chair or standing for extended periods but that improves after rest is a red flag for a posture-related condition.

Neck pain that continues into the upper back or into the lower back is also an indicator. Pain that radiates into the arms or legs is a more serious indicator of an advancing condition and should not be ignored. However, should the symptoms alleviate or lessen after switching positions, posture deficiencies should certainly be evaluated.

If you begin new activities that include extended sitting or standing and experience pain, or if you acquire a new chair, shoes, or workstation and pain sets in, that may also indicate a condition related to poor posture or poor mechanics. Pain that comes and goes for months is generally linked to postural strain and may be activity-related.

Get Up and Move

Not moving is more common in jobs that require you to sit most of the time. Driving doesn't exactly involve a lot of movement. If you were to become engrossed in a computer project, you might move your fingers on the keyboard but not much else.

Not moving leads to muscle fatigue. As the muscles fatigue, it becomes easier for your body to revert to poor postural positions, such as slouching and slumping. Maintaining these positions for extended periods puts additional pressure on the spine.

Movement is your key to reducing fatigue. Taking regular breaks (*at least one per hour*) will return blood flow to the muscles and help keep them from getting tired. There are software programs out there designed to monitor your posture, but a simple timer can help you remember to get up and move.

Regular exercise such as walking, swimming, or bicycling will help the body stay aerobically conditioned, while specific strengthening exercises will help the muscles surrounding the back to stay strong. These benefits of exercise promote good posture, which will, in turn, further help to condition muscles and prevent injury.

There are also specific exercises that will help you maintain good posture. In particular, a balance of trunk strength where the back muscles are about 30 percent stronger than the abdominal muscles is essential to help support the upper body and maintain good posture.

You can move while sitting by:

- ⮑ Rolling your shoulders
- ⮑ Stretching your neck
- ⮑ Tapping your toes

You can move while standing by:

- ⮑ Reaching overhead
- ⮑ Exaggerating some deep breaths

- ⊃ Stretching your arms behind you
- ⊃ Tapping your toes
- ⊃ Bending your knees
- ⊃ Performing "mini" lunges

Keep Your Body Straight

Keep your body as straight – or "neutral" – as possible, particularly when sitting in your office chair or standing for extended periods. You may have evaluated your posture from side to side, but you also need to keep your body weight distributed evenly from front to back. The more neutral your position, the less strain and pressure you put on your entire body.

Walking, lifting heavy materials, holding a telephone, and typing are all moving activities that require attention to ergonomics and posture. It is important to maintain good posture even while moving to avoid injury. Back injuries are especially common while twisting and/or lifting and often occur because of awkward movements and control of the upper body weight alone.

Avoid regularly wearing high-heeled shoes, which can affect the body's center of gravity and change the alignment of the entire body, negatively impacting back support and posture.

Use Posture Supports When Needed

Many people use posture supports as a posture "fix," even though this is not the intended purpose of the posture support. This is not to say that supports and aids are not useful (*although we will say that we think they are overused and can become an unnecessary crutch*). Posture aids are particularly useful if the ergonomic chair or work area is not totally supportive of your spine.

It makes sense that even the best ergonomic chair cannot possibly properly accommodate everyone from five feet tall to six-foot-seven.

There has to be some way to help the chair provide adequate support for everyone, even if it means adding stuff.

Footrests, portable lumbar back supports, or even a towel or small pillow can be used while sitting in an office chair and while driving. These are the types of posture supports you should consider.

When standing for long periods of time, placing a rubber mat on the floor can improve comfort. This will give your body more support and make it more likely that you will be able to maintain a healthy stance for a long period of time.

STANDING POSTURE

When people think about their posture, they notice it more when they're seated, and they believe their sitting posture is 100 percent responsible for the state of their neck and back. This is incorrect.

All the different posture positions – how you stand, sit, sleep, drive – how you do anything – affect your spine and overall posture. People seem to be less aware of what constitutes a bad posture position when standing, but it's the one they want to get right. They want to look and feel their best when standing.

Along these lines, when standing, we advise the following:

- ➲ Hold your head up straight with your chin in. Do not tilt your head forward, backward, or sideways.
- ➲ The bottoms of your ears should be in line with the middle of your shoulders.
- ➲ Keep your shoulder blades back.
- ➲ Keep your chest forward.
- ➲ Keep your knees straight (*but not locked*).
- ➲ Keep your weight evenly distributed on each leg; do not lean on one leg.

⊃ Tuck your stomach in. Do not tilt your pelvis forward or backward.

⊃ Make sure your shoes have good arch support or wear orthotics.

STANDING-DESK POSTURE

Use of a standing desk requires a combination of standing posture and computer posture. Using a standing desk has gotten much more popular, and for good reason. Sitting all day isn't good for you; having the option to stand is beneficial for your health.

However, people mistake a standing desk for "working on their posture." You can still have bad posture while using a standing desk as the benefits of using a standing desk are related more to the long-term negative effects of sitting, not bad posture. You still need to make sure you set up your standing desk to give you the best chance for good posture.

You want to do all the things you would do to have good standing posture, plus the following:

⊃ Adjust the height of the worktable to a comfortable level.

⊃ Try to elevate one foot by resting it on a stool or box. After several minutes, switch feet and elevate the other one.

⊃ Stand on a cushioned mat to decrease strain on your knees and back.

⊃ Make sure your monitor height is elevated, bringing the top of the monitor higher than eye level.

SITTING POSTURE

We can't tell you how many people think how silly it is to have to tell people how to sit. After all, how hard is it? Well, it must be very difficult because we hardly ever see anyone doing it right.

First of all, sit up! Your back should be straight with your shoulders back. Your butt should touch the back of your chair. (*Many people sit on the front of the chair's seat, totally eliminating the usefulness of the back of the chair.*) Always think tall! Think of a string that goes through your spine and up through your head. Then picture someone pulling you up by this string.

Ever so gently, pull yourself up by this string. With your shoulders back, allow your chest to open up fully. Take in full breaths, and think of the vitality and creativity that can come from better air flow to your body and your brain.

If absolutely necessary, use a back support (*even a small, rolled-up towel*) for your low back if the chair doesn't provide adequate support. Try to distribute your weight evenly between your hips.

Your knees should be bent at a ninety-degree angle. It's best if you can sit with your knees even with or slightly lower than your hips. This takes a lot of strain off the hips. Do not cross your legs (*this alone keeps most people from having good sitting posture!*), and keep your feet flat on the floor.

One last thing: don't sit on your wallet! I know this can be difficult, but it's the equivalent of walking with one shoe on all day or sitting on a block of wood. Either buy a smaller wallet and keep it in your front pocket, or keep your monster wallet and take it out when you sit (*including when driving*).

A long time ago, we had a recurring conversation with a patient who had one of the largest wallets we'd ever seen. This wallet had to be several inches thick, and the patient drove all day for his job. He didn't want to give up his wallet, but he was also tired of his back pain. His solution? He bought two giant wallets. It wasn't the most attractive solution, but it got the job done. Really, it's about keeping your body at neutral angles and as balanced as possible.

SMARTPHONE POSTURE

You're going to be on your phone, so let's do as little damage as possible while you're on it. Holding your phone down or on your lap is not required. You can hold your phone up in front of you or put it on something that is closer to eye level.

Remember, your head weighs about ten pounds. Looking down puts a lot of strain on the back of your neck, the back of your head, and your upper back. The more you do it, the longer those muscles get and the harder it is to change.

Limiting time on your phone would be the best way to maintain good posture. The next best way is to hold your phone up.

SLEEPING POSTURE

"What's the best way to sleep?" is probably the most common question our patients ask, and we're amazed by how many stomach sleepers are still out there. With all the strain we put on our necks all day, why do the same thing at night?

It's really not good to sleep on your stomach. As reformed stomach sleepers, we understand your pain (*literally!*). Sleeping on your stomach can lead to a great deal of low-back and neck pain before you finally make the change.

The first problem with sleeping on your stomach has to do with your neck. Since your bed is most likely not outfitted with a slot for your nose, you can either sleep facedown and have trouble breathing, or you can turn your head to one side.

Stomach sleepers are easy to identify by this one trait alone. You can likely turn your head very well to the side you turn it when you sleep, but only about 50 percent to the other side. This is a problem all by itself!

Turning your head to one side just a few times does not cause pain; it's about doing it repeatedly and for extended periods. Turning your head to one side while placing pressure on it for hours and hours every single night can lead to a problem that affects your neck vertebrae all the way down to the vertebrae of your upper back.

The next problem is with your lower back.

When lying face down, the muscles of your thigh push up the lower aspect of your back, forcing your lumbar spine into hyperextension – that is, too much curve. The bones jam up on themselves and increase the likelihood of low-back pain.

A similar situation occurs in your lower back as it does in your neck. While lying facedown for a moment doesn't cause a problem, lying in that position for hours will eventually lead to a low-back problem and then pain.

Making the change from being a stomach sleeper to a back sleeper is often a very difficult transition. Even if you start out on your back, you probably won't stay that way. Throw in the fact that you are significantly more likely to start snoring when you are sleeping on your back, and your partner may make the change even more difficult. (*It's hard to become a back sleeper when you're getting poked and shoved all night as your partner hisses, "Roll over! You're snoring loud enough to wake the neighbors!"*)

The next best way of sleeping is sleeping on your side, which is the easiest transition to make if you are a chronic stomach sleeper. To begin to take the most pressure off your spine, you need to do a couple things. As always, we recommend involving a helper to take a look at your sleeping position. The most comfortable position is not always the best for you. (*By the way, your helper doesn't have to come over at bedtime and watch you sleep. Just lie down in your bed during the day, fully clothed with the lights on, and have them take a look.*)

Next, let's examine your pillow. Ideally, your head should remain straight while on the pillow. It should not dip down into a pillow that's too soft or be propped up because your pillow is too thick and/or firm. It's almost always a bad idea to have more than one pillow (*unless they're paper-thin*). Your head should be positioned at a ninety-degree angle to your shoulder, nice and straight.

A pillow between your knees is also essential. Your hips and knees will thank you for taking the pressure off. The best choice for this is a body pillow. It gives you something to grab onto, mimics some of the things you probably liked about sleeping on your stomach, and is long enough for you to have a pillow between your knees. Since you are holding it, it will move with you should you roll over.

(*We've seen pillows that strap onto your leg, keeping them from getting "lost" in the middle of the night. This isn't the most attractive thing we've ever seen, and we've wondered what would happen in case of a fire. There you are, running from your home with a pillow strapped to your leg …*)

The idea behind using a body pillow is to limit any rotation of your pelvis and, therefore, your lumbar spine. Pull the pillow firmly against your body, with your top leg on the pillow and your ankle and foot supported on it too. Your upper body should have the top arm wrapped around the pillow so that there's no rotation of the upper back.

The only drawback to the body pillow is that it's so big! It can be like adding an additional person in the bed. The trade-off is well worth it, though, and many stores sell these giant pillows. They are easy to find for a reasonable price.

What is the best way to sleep?

So you've finally decided to sleep on your back? Good for you – as long as you don't snore, or even if you do and you sleep by yourself. Sleeping on your back should be the easiest way to keep your spine in good alignment for six to eight hours each night.

We know sleeping sounds simple. Lie on your back. Go to sleep. Wake up. What else is there? … A lot!

Let's keep in mind that we want to keep your spine in the best position possible when you sleep. If nothing else, this should keep you from continuing to damage your spine each night, even if it's not necessarily fixing anything.

The best way to sleep is on your back with a pillow under your knees and a pillow under your head and neck that is supportive without pushing your head up. If you can't do that, sleeping on your side with a pillow between your knees (*or a body pillow*) and a pillow under your head that lets you keep a neutral spine is second-best.

You should not be sleeping on your stomach if you hope to have good posture long-term.

If you are a stomach sleeper, we suggest switching to sleeping on your side. If you use a body pillow, you can hug it and still get that "snuggly" feeling you get when sleeping on your stomach – but without twisting your head. We have not seen many patients successfully make the transition from stomach sleeping to back sleeping. You really have to be committed to make that change, and the aggravation probably isn't worth it.

Visit our website at https://www.betterposturefast.com/step1 for a video demonstrating the right sleeping posture.

> **BETTER POSTURE TIP:** Stop sleeping on your stomach as soon as possible! You likely won't make it all the way to your back, but being a side sleeper is the next best option. Your neck and upper back will thank you right away, and your lower back will thank you over time.

DRIVING POSTURE

If you spend a lot of time in the car, you have to pay attention to how you're sitting. Sitting on your wallet, sitting with one leg up on the seat, or leaning into the middle console will put your spine in a bad position, and you won't even realize you're doing it.

Keeping your hair in a ponytail when driving for extended periods is also not recommended. That ponytail tends to push your head forward and can lead to neck strain followed by headaches at the back of your head. It's all about keeping your position as neutral as possible.

For good driving posture:

- ⮀ Use a back support (*lumbar roll*) at the curve of your back. You can use a posture support or a small towel rolled up with rubber bands to keep it in place. If you've seen a chiropractor that takes X-rays, you will know if you have too much spinal curve or too little. This can help you determine the size of the support you should get.
- ⮀ Your knees should be at the same level or higher than your hips. If the knees are lower than the hips, the angle between the spine and the thighs increases. This begins to increase stress on your lower back.
- ⮀ Move the seat close to the steering wheel to support the curve of your back (*without being so close that you are worried about what would happen if the airbag deployed*). The seat should be close enough to allow your knees to be in the proper position (*as described above*) and your feet to reach the pedals.
- ⮀ Your elbows should be in a relaxed bend of about twenty degrees. Your upper back, shoulders, and neck should be relaxed. You should be able to take in deep breaths and calmly focus on your driving.

COMPUTER POSTURE

People often ask us about proper computer posture, and we regularly speak about this topic at companies. There are plenty of diagrams, workstations, and chairs claiming to be the answer to your computer-posture issues.

Some companies have ergonomic experts that come and take measurements and help employees find an optimal workstation, but this isn't the most common scenario.

Your computer posture should be an extension of the exercises you are already doing to improve your posture. Your computer posture should not be taking away from the good work you're doing to improve your posture.

YOUR CHAIR

Before you go out and spend a lot of money on the top-of-the-line chair, double-check your workstation and make sure that you've covered all the bases there. Saying your chair can make or break your posture is not totally true because you must exercise to have good posture. Getting a chair to fix your posture will only lead to frustration. Your chair should support your good posture to help you maintain what you've worked on.

Still, too many people think that they can passively improve their posture by buying the "right" chair, and that is just not true! Select your chair with the idea that you will be diligently working on improving your posture through exercise, and then you will steadily improve your surroundings to support your efforts.

We are not all the same height and weight, nor do we all sit at the same workstation for the same lengths of time. This is why we can't just say, "Go buy Chair A, and good posture is yours!" That would be nice, but it's not possible. However, knowing what you're looking for and what to avoid, combined with your budget, will help you get the most out of your selection.

Here are the most important things to consider:

- ➲ The chair must be height adjustable.
- ➲ The armrests must be height adjustable.
- ➲ With your buttocks against the back of the chair, attempt to pass a clenched fist between the front of your chair and the back of your calf. If you can't do that, the chair is too deep for you.
- ➲ If the chair is too deep, you can try to adjust its backrest and move it forward or insert a lumbar support.
- ➲ The chair's backrest must be adjustable.
- ➲ The chair should offer lumbar support (*low-back support*).
- ➲ The chair's material should breathe (*cloth instead of a hard surface*).
- ➲ The chair should swivel (*rotate*).
- ➲ The chair should have a rounded front edge (*allows for better circulation*).

Just like when you choose a mattress, you're going to have to check out the chairs because you can rule out a lot sitting in them in the store. First, you have to consider what you do during your day. Are you primarily on your keyboard or your mouse? Do you have a large workspace to cover? (*This can make a difference in the type of wheels or casters you choose.*) Many people read a guide and say, "My chair has to fit this way and that way," but they forget that they don't really use their chair that way.

Do you lean back in your chair a lot? How much space is available to accommodate this super-chair you're going to buy? Are you accepting the recommendation of someone half your size – or twice your size?

YOUR KEYBOARD AND MOUSE

Your mouse and keyboard should be at the same height.

Keeping your mouse and keyboard at the same height and preferably near each other minimizes the posture changes you have to make each time you switch from one to the other.

Your wrists should be straight.

Keeping your wrists straight (*neutral*) reduces the risk of repetitive stress (*strain*) injury (*RSI*). If your wrists are forced to bend up, down, or to the side while you use your keyboard and mouse, you increase the likelihood that you will develop wrist problems, including carpal tunnel syndrome.

Your keyboard should be at the same height as your elbows.

This will keep your forearms level and your wrists neutral. It also means that you cannot keep your keyboard on top of your desk! Keyboard trays can be easily installed to bring your keyboard down to a non-damaging level.

You should be able to reach all the keys without straining.

This may be getting a little picky, but you should be able to easily reach all the keys of your keyboard. Everyone is not the same size! Thankfully, there are now smaller keyboards available to help with this. This is just one more thing to consider when looking for every possible way to keep yourself from developing problems from your everyday activities.

Remember, sometimes the smallest things lead to some of the biggest problems when that small thing is repeated over and over and over again.

YOUR MONITORS

Your monitor (or monitors) should be directly in front of you.

Okay, pretty obvious, right? Nope. We still have to tell our patients to do this. You should not have to turn your neck to look at your monitor while typing. This happens most often when you've put your monitor in the corner of the desk. You should strive to get everything straight in front of you as much as possible.

When using two monitors, people will have one of two setups: one screen in front and one to the side, or both in front and side by side. If you have one screen in front of you, that means you have to turn your head to use the other screen. We know it can be awkward, but your neck and spine will thank you if you move that side monitor from one side to the other every month. Let the start of the new month be your reminder to move your second screen from the right side of your desk to the left.

Putting both monitors in front of you seems like a great way to beat the system, but you'll still end up with a dominant screen. Let's say your email is always on the right screen and your spreadsheets are always on the left. Chances are you'll spend more of your day on one screen than the other. Use the first of the month as your reminder to switch what's on the screens. Move your email to the left monitor and your spreadsheets to the right.

It may seem like a small change, but spending forty to fifty hours per week like this can really add up. Good posture is built on consistency, and the more balanced and consistent you can keep your activities, the longer you'll maintain good posture.

Your eyes should be about two feet from the monitor.

If your monitor is very large, you may have to move back a little more. This again seems like an easy one, but with the invention of the wireless keyboard, people are zooming all over the place in their chairs and keeping their monitors in strange places.

One of our patients utilized his optometrist to help him get glasses that are only in focus when he's in good posture and the right distance away. If he starts to slouch, his screen isn't as clear. It's an easy (*but, according to him, sometimes annoying*) way to make sure you're sitting with good posture.

At a minimum, your eyes should be level with the top of the monitor.

Ideally, you should be able to look slightly down to see the middle of the screen. You should not have to lean your head back or forward to see your monitor. If your monitor height is adjustable, this should be an easy step for you. If not, you can use a book or another handy object to get your monitor to a good level.

Even better, put the top of your monitor higher than eye level. If you can slouch and still see your screen easily, you will do that. If maintaining a good position makes your setup ideal, even better.

If you fix nothing else with your computer posture, fix the height and position of your monitors. You can get a lot of stuff wrong, but you can't miss this one. So many patients end their headaches and neck pain quickly by making just this one change.

YOUR LAPTOP

We don't think there's a perfect way to use your laptop because you're going to have to sacrifice something. If you actually put the laptop on your lap while sitting in a chair, you're slumping.

If you put the laptop on top of your desk, you will sacrifice your wrists, but you can save your neck and back. It's okay to work in either of these positions for a short time, but that's not what people do with their laptops.

Ideally, you should use your laptop more like a monitor by raising it up on books or a stand. Then you can purchase an external keyboard and mouse to get your arms and wrists into the right positions. You could also plug your laptop into an external monitor at home and use your laptop more like a keyboard.

TIPS FOR WORKING FROM HOME

As we write this book, a huge portion of the population now works from home. Having never worked from home for this long before, people have found their ergonomic setup at home to be less than desirable.

At their office, they've got a sit/stand desk and a good chair. Maybe an ergonomic expert even arrived to measure them to make sure their work space is set up correctly. At home, they're sitting on the couch with their laptop on their legs, looking down at their monitors for hours. Others are lying in bed with their laptop or sitting at the dining table in chairs "barely comfortable to sit in during a meal" (*according to one of our patients*).

If you find yourself working at home and want to save your spine and your posture but have a limited budget, your best investment is to buy a larger monitor or a stand that will raise your laptop screen to a higher level.

You cannot have good posture with a laptop unless you raise that screen, forcing you to sit up straighter. However, when we discuss with patients how they're fixing their home setup, they almost always talk about getting a better chair. A chair is great and will help your lower back, but raising your screen will force you into a better posture position.

Yes, you should be looking at the height of your desk or table. Yes, you should make sure your office chair provides some level of support. However, if you get the monitor set up correctly, you will save yourself a lot of pain and spinal damage.

Since you're at home, setting a timer and stretching every hour is much more easily accomplished. Stretch your neck, go through all your spinal ranges of motion, and walk around a bit. We've included a bunch of exercises on our website at https://www.betterposturefast.com/step2.

> **BETTER POSTURE TIP:** It can be a challenge to fix everything with your computer setup, and you may have limited options. If you can fix only one thing, make sure you raise your monitor or screen height. This will force you into good posture for longer periods of time.

YOUR MATTRESS

A common scenario in our office is the arrival of a new patient complaining of low-back pain. "What have you done about it so far?" I ask.

"Well, the first thing I did was go out and buy the best mattress I could. I figured my back hurt because my bed wasn't right."

While this is not an illogical conclusion, our next question seems to floor them. "How did you know you were getting the right mattress for you?"

"I, uh, …bought the best one!"

Just about every mattress company offers different versions of their mattresses. They aren't selling the "This will hurt your back" model vs. the "This won't hurt your back" model.

Some of the lower-priced mattress options may be just right for some people. How do you decide? It seems there's a lot of confusion out there, so if you're in this boat, you're definitely not alone.

Given that the average person spends one-third of their life in bed (*approximately*), you would be surprised to find out there has been little scientific research performed on mattresses.

THE FOUNDATION

We'll get to the mattress portion of the bed in a minute, but let's quickly discuss the foundation of your bed, also known as the box spring. The box spring supports the mattress and is comparable to the shock absorbers in your car.

Many people ignore the benefits of a box spring and either eliminate it from their setup or put their good mattress on the floor. The foundation can have springs (*that's why they call it a "box spring"*) or no springs.

The springs distribute your weight more evenly across its frame for better wear and tear. The benefit of the weight distribution can be outweighed by the possibility that your box spring will "squeak."

Foam mattresses typically utilize a wooden frame as springs are not needed. (*Foam foundations are available for the foam mattresses and should not be used with coiled-spring mattresses.*) The wooden frames are made of different grades of wood that do not necessarily affect your ability to sleep, but which do impact their lifespan. Obviously cheaper wood will wear faster and lose their supportive effect sooner.

Mixing and matching your mattress and foundations is not recommended. This can lead to incomplete support, reducing the effectiveness of your investment. Also, the mixing and matching may void your warranty (*particularly if you are putting a new mattress on an old box spring*).

A quality mattress should last you between eight and ten years. Combine that with your comfort and desire to avoid back problems, and you've got quite a decision on your hands. We will provide you with some concepts to keep in mind when choosing your new mattress, but if you follow all these suggestions and still aren't comfortable with the bed, please don't continue to use it! The better mattress companies usually offer at least a sixty-night guarantee, and it may take the entire sixty nights for you to decide if you've chosen correctly.

Your doctor can offer some suggestions (*or things to avoid*) if you have a specific condition. Also, if you have a very similar body type as a family member and they are thrilled with their bed, you have another leg up on making your decision. (*And if they didn't like a particular bed, this added information can be very helpful too.*)

BUYING NEW

Considering even the best mattress should be replaced every ten years, how much available use are you getting by purchasing a used bed? Probably not a whole lot. The mattress may look fine, but the core of the mattress is probably ready for a change. After all, why were they getting rid of it?

Other issues when buying a used mattress are the possibility the mattress contains dust mites or other pests and/or may not meet updated safety standards. Remember, you will be spending one-third of your life on this thing. Don't buy a used mattress if you can avoid it.

DETERMINE THE SIZE OF YOUR MATTRESS

If we had to summarize this section in one sentence, it would be "Bigger is better." Keep in mind that your bed will need to fit in your bedroom. Other than that, get the biggest bed you can afford. The extra room will increase your and/or your partner's comfort.

This next tip may seem obvious, but it is often overlooked: try out the bed! Some people get caught up in thinking they can't simulate their sleep environment, so they don't think about trying out beds in public or during the day. If you and your partner will be sleeping on the bed each night, go to the store together and try it out.

The more things you can rule out and not leave to chance, the more likely you'll be successful in choosing your bed.

MATTRESS FIRMNESS

We have heard people say for years that when they had issues with their mattress or their back, they went out and bought the firmest mattress they could buy. "I bought the best mattress I could get – it's so firm!" The results, however, were always mixed.

Some people would be happy they got the firm mattress, while others had to return it. Firm mattresses have been prescribed for years by many medical professionals (*but not chiropractors*), though there wasn't a lot of research behind this advice. The underlying philosophy was that while the soft mattress feels good, it doesn't provide much support. How to know for sure?

Technology has advanced now to the point that you can adjust the firmness of your bed, varying the result between you and your partner. Still, are you getting the best support? Finally, more research has become available.

A research study out of Spain used 313 patients with a history of low-back pain and gave them firm and medium-firm mattresses. All the participants had previously complained of feeling pain in their lower backs when lying in bed and when they were getting out of bed. The participants were not told which bed they were using for the study. The group with the medium-firm mattresses reported improvements in their low-back pain twice as often as those on the firm mattresses.

Some believe the study may be a bit skewed by the idea that the patients included may have simply needed a new mattress. Many people don't change their mattresses as often as recommended, or they purchase a used mattress that has already passed its usefulness period.

Still, would you be the person that reported improvement with the firm mattress? Only a handful of studies report improvements with a firm mattress, but since there is little research overall, it is difficult to determine. Also, research often only provides the information for categories like "more likely" or "twice as likely"; rarely do we get anything that says "always."

We have learned in practice that there are therapies that work best for most people, but rarely is there anything that works across the board with every patient with every condition. Much of this is trial and error; we start with the most logical conclusion and move on from there.

We want to help you get to your most logical conclusion, but you need to realize you are going to have to try out the mattresses until you arrive at the right conclusion for you. As such, it's usually best to find a store with a liberal policy for trying out the bed. We recommend never purchasing a bed from a company that won't let you use it for at least a thirty-day trial period (*most will allow longer*).

Surveys have indicated that orthopedic doctors continue to recommend firm mattresses to their patients anywhere from two out of three, to three out of four times. Chiropractors have long recommended that this may not be the right choice.

Chiropractors have traditionally recommended a medium-firm mattress with the addition of a layer of padding that is one and a half to two inches thick. The philosophy behind this is that the extra padding allows for a more evenly dispersed support to better adapt to the normal curvatures of the spine.

The additional padding is usually available where you buy your mattress and from other stores that sell bedding supplies.

COILED-SPRING MATTRESS

The coiled-spring mattress is the most common type on the market today, and it's also the type to which most people have become accustomed. There are two types – continuous and independent.

In a continuous-spring mattress, each coil is an ongoing part of one system. The advantage of this type of mattress is that it makes the mattress less likely to begin sagging in one place. The disadvantage is that the system cannot be responsive to the individual shape of your body. (*You also can't jump on one side without spilling a glass of wine on the other side – per a popular commercial.*)

Independent-coil mattress systems utilize coils that are separate (*as the name suggests*) to give more flexible support across the individual sections of your body. These systems are more expensive, and those that opt for a cheap version can be disappointed when the coils give way quickly. In addition, since more stress can be put on an individual coil, there may be uneven wear and tear.

The total number of coils is also typically indicative of the quality of the mattress. However, no specific number of coils has been determined to be the best. It's simply true that the more coils, the firmer the mattress.

As we've discussed, if the mattress is too firm, it may not be the most ideal mattress for you. If the mattress has fewer coils (*more common in cheaper mattresses*), it will be less firm, but it will also put more strain on the coils.

AIR MATTRESS

Okay, we're not recommending that you sleep on a raft you used in your swimming pool. Even the inflatable beds used by unfortunate guests are not likely to provide the right kind of support you need (*as evidenced by the soreness in your back on your last visit to the in-laws*).

We're talking about the mattresses that use inflatable air chambers to adjust firmness with a remote control. For example, the Sleep Number bed assigns you a number based on a "pressure mapping" system that uses a computer to determine which level of firmness is best for you.

These beds are good for couples because they have two separate chambers, enabling your partner to have an entirely different number than you. This is particularly useful if you need a firm mattress and your partner needs something totally different.

Although we've heard mostly good things about these beds, the complaints we've heard from dissatisfied customers have to do with the bed not being as comfortable as they would like. In particular, the air chamber is surrounded by padding, and it's possible to roll off the air chamber portion and into the edging. This issue seems to be more prevalent in the lower-end models.

We tried an air mattress with a pillow top and were unable to find the air chamber or the hard edge mentioned by others. The mattress makers of this model work hard to make sure you've got the right level of support, as having an adjustable mattress doesn't do you any good if you're on the wrong setting.

Finding out your "sleep number" can give you insight into the level of firmness that is right for you. We regularly advise patients to start their search at these stores because they get so much information about the right level of firmness they need for their body type.

FOAM MATTRESS

Originally developed by NASA to help astronauts deal with the enormous g-forces experienced during takeoff, the material has now been put to use in our mattresses. The idea is that if the foam can absorb the forces of gravity during takeoff, surely it can help support you during sleep.

The "memory" foam absorbs your body heat and molds itself to the contours of your body to support you as needed. The foam is also beneficial for couples, as it adapts to them individually. This can be particularly useful if one partner is significantly larger than the other.

One drawback we've heard is that if you tend to get hot while you sleep, the material is more likely to exaggerate your body heat rather than help dissipate it. In other words, if you get hot sleeping on a spring mattress, expect that you'll get hotter sleeping on a foam mattress.

If this is not a concern for you (*maybe you're always cold*), then this mattress may be the right choice for you. These mattresses are typically not cheap, but they are certainly catching on, gaining support from medical experts and chiropractors who are pleased with the spinal support offered. The foam allows your hips and shoulders to sink into the bed while supporting your waist and legs.

Currently there is no truly significant research to support any of these claims, though they do seem to make logical sense. People that own these types of beds say that it takes some time to adjust to them since they don't feel as plush as what they may be used to.

"Mattress experts" recommend that your memory foam mattress include a minimum of 4-5 cm of foam to properly provide the support you are seeking. If you can't afford a memory foam mattress or want to upgrade your current mattress, you may consider adding a foam mattress topper.

SUMMARY

You should get a new mattress every eight to ten years. Most mattresses include warranties that last from ten to fifteen years, but that's for the mattress – not your level of support or comfort.

Mattress manufacturers typically recommend that you rotate your mattress at least twice per year, but every three months is best. The goal is to reduce – or eliminate completely – any sagging or indentations in your sleeping area. If you start sinking into the bed, this can lead to back problems.

Overall, you're going to want a mattress that's not too hard and not too soft; you want one that is right for you. It may seem that we're dancing around the subject, but our bodies are not made equally. We personally have relatives that happily sleep on the floor to help their back, something that would leave us incapacitated for days.

Think about what you want this mattress to do. You want all your key spinal areas to be supported while gravity does its thing on you while you're asleep. If your mattress were super-firm (*like made out of metal*), it would have no "give" to it, and your shoulder would be compressed, bearing the entire force of your weight while you slept on your side.

If your bed were super-soft and you slept on your side, your shoulders and hips would bear the entire pressure. However, the unsupported points on your spine would begin to sag. The sagging every night would put extra stress on your spine, pulling it out of alignment and stressing the ligaments and joints of the spine.

The ideal scenario would be to find a mattress that conforms to your pressure points while providing adequate support to the natural curves of your spine. Finding this ideal scenario is going to require some trial and error. That's why we recommend working with a local store (*if possible*) that offers a liberal return policy if you're not happy or if it's just not the right bed for you.

We will recommend, however, that you steer clear of the spring mattresses. Their time has come and gone, and there are better alternatives available. The people who sell air beds that assign you a number have a great device that "pressure maps" where you are putting your weight when you lie down, and they use this information to assign the right firmness for you. Other stores are now catching on with similar technology to help you with a better starting point to finding the right mattress for you.

We think the foam mattress is going to give great support to most people for their posture issues. Other than getting warm, the responses I've heard from patients seem to give this the best chance for your success.

> **BETTER POSTURE TIP:** While having a good mattress is important, it likely shouldn't be the first thing you spend money on if you develop neck and lower-back pain. Very often your sleeping position or your pillow height is a greater contributor to your pain.

YOUR PILLOW

You've chosen the perfect mattress for yourself, but your neck still hurts. This is very often related to your sleep posture and your pillow. We have some patients with a closet full of pillows that just don't work for them.

If you're a back sleeper, we recommend that you use a pillow with support for your neck. You shouldn't be sleeping on more than one pillow, as that would push your neck forward.

Patients that have tried the special neck-support pillows and didn't like them usually had the wrong size. Pillow manufacturers often provide different sizes and sizing charts, so take advantage of this information. These pillows are definitely not one-size-fits-all.

If you're a side sleeper, you do not need a curved neck-support pillow. You need a pillow that fills the space between your neck and shoulder. The side-sleeping pillow will be larger than the back-sleeping pillow. A firmer, foam-type pillow usually works great for keeping that space consistent and not allowing your neck to tilt one way or the other. Neutral angles are best, keeping your head at ninety degrees to your shoulder. It is worth measuring the distance from one side of your neck to the outer edge of your shoulder to see how big your pillow should be.

We also recommend a big body pillow for side sleepers. This gives you something to hug, which will keep your shoulders in a more neutral position, and it can also fit between your knees. This keeps your shoulders from jamming up during the night and adding shoulder pain to your list of problems.

There isn't a right pillow for stomach sleepers because you shouldn't be doing that! A current list of pillows we recommend for our patients is available for your review at https://www.betterposturefast/resources.

▶ CHAPTER 7

POSTURE SUPPORTS & GADGETS

Posture supports, braces, and gadgets are a booming industry, and they all claim to fix all your neck and back pain problems. We have found that some are helpful, and some don't do much of anything. None of them will "fix" bad posture; they will only support, enhance, or minimize some issues. You'll still need to add in stretches, exercises, and (*likely*) a visit to a chiropractor to see lasting changes.

Posture gadgets fall into one of the following categories: braces, supports, traction devices, or reminding devices.

POSTURE BRACES

This may be the most controversial part of this book. Most of the patients I encounter seem to think that they can just strap their shoulders back and their posture problem will be solved. This is a common – and very dangerous – misunderstanding. The only thing saving most people is that they wear their posture supports so inconsistently that they never have a chance to suffer the complications.

Here's an example: In an attempt to lower the prevalence of back injuries suffered from heavy lifting, a local home-improvement store issued back braces to all their employees. The employees immediately began wearing the back braces … the entire time they were on the job.

There was nothing inherently wrong with the back brace. It was a good back brace, it fit well, and it supported the spine and the muscles of the low back well. So what's the problem? What is the potential danger of wearing the back brace all the time?

You've heard the phrase "use it or lose it." Regarding your posture muscles, this is absolutely true. If you are not using your muscles (*because they are in a brace all day*), they get weaker – and it's not the kind of weakness you're going to notice right away. Your muscles are getting increasingly weaker and weaker, but you keep putting on the brace and heading to work.

With the use of these back braces over time, the number of back injuries increased at the home-improvement store, instead of decreasing. How is this possible? At the start of the back-brace use, the muscles were stronger. Then they began to weaken as they were supported by the brace.

After a while, the braces were supporting weaker and weaker backs until, eventually, the braces were the only things holding everything together. The back injuries occurred not necessarily while lifting something, but during activities that shouldn't cause a back injury, like picking up a piece of paper off the floor (*when not wearing the brace*).

You'll still see these braces in use at this home-improvement store, with one additional twist. They are loose around the employee's waist until it's time to lift something. Then the employee tightens the brace, lifts the object, and then returns the brace to its loose position.

Understanding this example, what do you think will happen to you if you have something strapped around your shoulders day in and day out? Will your shoulders and supporting muscles get stronger? Not in a million years.

We certainly understand why someone would seek out a posture brace. The pictures make it seem like it's going to work fine. Put one on, and your posture will look significantly better … for a short time.

We recommend braces in crisis only – for example, if you hurt your lower back and need the brace to keep you out of pain. Patients won't typically need to wear the brace for more than a week or two in these situations. The goal is to get them out of the brace as quickly as possible.

Another example would be patients dealing with compression fractures associated with the dowager's hump. In this case, the extreme nature of their osteoporosis and the pain of the spinal fracture mean they definitely need an increase in support. The brace may be needed for a much longer time to help prevent additional fractures, to allow the current fracture to heal, and to decrease the pain level associated with the fracture.

For reviews of posture braces and feedback on the best ones, visit https://www.betterposturefast/resources.

POSTURE SUPPORTS

In contrast with posture braces, posture supports like a good chair or good shoes are worth considering. However, the changes the supports are attempting to make should not be drastic. They should be there to help remind you and even to prevent you from assuming a bad postural position, but not to correct the position.

You should definitely consider using a low-back support in your car while driving (*especially if you drive for considerable distances and your seat does not come with a built-in lumbar-support feature*).

Good pillows and proper support while you sleep are also key (*and well covered in other areas of this book*).

The main conclusion here is that posture supports are designed to do just that – support. They are not the answer to your posture-correction needs. If the changes they are trying to make are too dramatic, they could do more harm than good.

Too many patients believe that by purchasing a "support" they are solving their problem, but this is just not the case. True posture changes can't be made by just using a support, but you can certainly make your posture worse by not using supports.

You may keep reading this book looking for an alternative to exercise as the way to change your posture, but you're not going to find it. How else are you going to get your muscles to support your body if you don't exercise them? Use supports to help your spine stay in a good position or to minimize strain, but don't think they're fixing your posture.

For a list of recommended supports for various types of activities, visit https://www.betterposturefast/resources.

POSTURE GADGETS THAT TRACTION

Lately, social media is filled with the newest version of neck or low-back traction. Traction has been around in one form or another for years. Why? Because it feels good and is good for you.

Some traction devices seem more barbaric than others, and some are just easier to use than others. They all work by pulling on your spine to create more space between your vertebrae. This is a good thing.

Traction may be achieved by someone or something pulling on your head, by hanging from a pull-up bar, by lying on the floor with your feet up on the couch, by using an inversion table, or by spinal decompression therapy. All of these do a specific action in the hope of achieving a similar result.

Some traction devices will pull a little, while others can pull with a lot more force. Some of the traction devices that hook to the door won't pull very hard, but you don't need a lot of force when it comes to your neck.

Inversion tables can work great, but you're still only getting what gravity can give you … and you have to be (*at least a little*) upside down.

Traction is a good thing when it comes to the health of your spine, and it can help free up movement in your spine to help you improve your posture. Once you find a traction device you like, consistency is key. Gravity is a constant force pulling you down, and traction pulls the other way. Gravity is going to win, but we can slow it down and help your spine and discs stay as healthy as possible.

For a list of recommended traction devices visit https://www.betterposturefast/resources.

POSTURE GADGETS THAT REMIND

Let us say this for the record: you cannot remind yourself enough to have good posture. You just can't. We've never seen our patients be successful using a reminding device, and we don't believe you will achieve Better Posture Fast using one either.

We've seen patients use sticky notes, smartphone apps, and various versions of "buzzing" gadgets that alert you to slouching or bad posture. There's a small chance you will sit up straight a few times, but no one we've spoken to was willing to get alerted all day long. We like the idea, and we can see why people look to these devices for help, but the way we'll show you to improve your posture won't require you to be constantly reminded.

► C H A P T E R   8

IMPROVE YOUR POSTURE PRACTITIONERS

Given that many bad-posture conditions are going to need a little extra help to correct, we've put together the most likely prospects you can use to help you achieve your posture goals. We stress again that if you do the exercises and watch your posture, you should do fine.

However, if you are not getting the results you want and you are concerned that you may have a condition that can't be fixed by exercise, these "improve your posture" practitioners have specialized areas that can be of assistance.

CHIROPRACTORS

Chiropractic can be very beneficial when your spine has become involved in your poor posture. If you hold an improper position too long, your spinal joints can become fixated or stuck in the wrong position.

In particular, if you are simply unable to stand up straight – your memory can no longer even get this done and you are stuck or locked in the forward-hunching position – it is time to visit a chiropractor because your bones are likely stuck and out of alignment. This is not something you should try to take care of yourself.

A chiropractic adjustment finds the area of your spine (*it's usually not the entire spine*) that is out of alignment and helps restore its normal position and function. That "pop" you might hear is your vertebra becoming unstuck. Yeah! (*There are also "non-popping" ways to move your spine, if you're afraid of the pops.*)

You can probably make your bones "pop" on your own, but please don't do it around us. Each vertebra can move out of place up to sixteen different ways. Unless you're a chiropractor, you likely have no idea which way it has moved, which means you have no idea the direction it needs to move to go back to its proper location. So don't do it! We don't adjust ourselves either. Luckily we work with great chiropractors (*and each other*), so great chiropractic care is always around.

When you have your friend bear-hug you at the family barbeque and lift you up and down, resulting in a chorus of "pops," you have not done a good thing. I know, I know, it feels better. The reason for that is the "pop" has released your body's own natural painkillers, called endorphins and enkephalins. These substances are released even when the vertebra is moved the wrong way, and even if the vertebra you moved didn't need to move in the first place.

Here's the way some people get their back "cracked" (*it gives us the chills*). They … let … other people … walk on their backs. Oops! Is that you? Please stop doing that too. Again, your spine is designed to move and function a specific way. Moving it the wrong way is not what we want.

When a chiropractor performs a chiropractic adjustment, they are not only moving the vertebra the right direction, they are moving only the one that needs to move! We use small bones in our hands or special instruments to accomplish this. Someone's foot is nowhere near as specific. How could it be? (*Not that the person doing the stomping has any idea which direction they were hoping to move the vertebra anyway.*)

Okay, so adjusting your own spine is bad. Letting a trained Doctor of Chiropractic do it is good. Once you've undergone a chiropractic treatment plan, you still need to do the exercises to keep your spine in good shape and your posture up to par.

Chiropractors can also help with some of the conditions we've indicated that you can't fix on your own. Your posture is the window to your spine – who better to take a look at your spine than a chiropractor?

In our office, we will likely take X-rays to see exactly what's going on in your spine and the direction vertebrae are out of alignment, and to look for anything that would modify how we take care of you. X-rays also let us know if it is safe to treat you.

This extra step also enables us to see structural changes over time. We believe it's important to get the right X-rays prior to starting chiropractic care, but not all chiropractic offices share this approach. Later in this book, we will share with you the exact method we use to evaluate our patients and why we feel getting on a plan is so important to your long-term results.

PHYSICAL THERAPISTS

If you don't think you can follow through with the exercises on your own, physical therapy may be a route to consider. Our goal is to see you have the best posture you can have for as long as possible. Sometimes you just need a jump start. You should know, though, that unless you get a referral from your physician and your insurance covers it, physical therapy will not be cheap.

However, part of the practice of physical therapy is to evaluate posture and create an exercise program to help correct what is needed. The physical therapist can use exercises, stretching, massage, and other muscle and soft-tissue techniques to accomplish this goal. They can also help you find exercises you can actually do. Some patients can't get up from the floor on their own, so the therapist can figure out a program that won't require any floor time.

Make sure you find a physical therapist that will provide "active" care instead of "passive" care like ultrasound and electric muscle stimulation. While passive care is great for new injuries, they will not help your posture. You're going to have to do active things (*like exercise*) to make a change.

The physical therapist is going to make you exercise. Hmm … where have you heard that before? The most beneficial part of physical therapy is that they assess which exercises you can and can't do and make modifications to help you progress.

We have provided good exercises and stretches and included some modifications to help you level up, but some people need to start even smaller. Physical therapists do a great job of giving you exercises you can do with any current physical limitations you may have and then building incrementally from there.

MASSAGE THERAPISTS

Massage can certainly help relax your muscles, but it is not going to strengthen them. In particular, the "relaxing" massage will likely do nothing to alleviate your posture issue.

With poor posture, certain muscles get overworked, causing them to fatigue, spasm, and then harden. Massage can relax these muscles, increase the blood flow to the area, and decrease the rate of degeneration.

Deep-tissue massage is going to be the most helpful technique. While this type of massage can be painful, the benefits will last much longer than the lighter, less intensive tissue massage. "No pain, no gain" is appropriate here.

Speaking of painful, a technique called Rolfing is also adept at making postural changes in the spine. Rolfers are not the easiest to find, but there is usually at least one practitioner in any major city.

A Rolfing "massage" is a deep-tissue massage on another level. Rolfing is referred to as "Structural Integration" by some practitioners. While we already discussed that a deep-tissue massage can be painful, this session will be as well. Since the practitioner is going deeper, the benefits will last even longer than a deep-tissue massage.

Practitioners who provide this type of massage are known as a "Rolfers." Named for the originator, Dr. Ida Rolf, Rolfers seek to align the entire body by manipulating the muscles and connective tissue of the spine. Our personal experience with Rolfing has been almost totally positive.

While the working of the fascia and connective tissue can be painful, the Rolfer shows you proper ways to breathe to eliminate the pain. The results are good and last a long time, although I did have one patient who sought out Rolfing while dealing with a severely inflamed low-back condition and just wasn't quite ready to undergo that type of treatment.

Rolfing starts with ten sessions designed to address the entire body as a whole. It's not truly a massage, as its approach is entirely different from what you may be used to. Still, if your body needs a major overhaul to get your posture going in the right direction, you should consider this.

And, yes, after that you still need to do the exercises!

YOGA

There is more to yoga than just getting more flexible. Yoga has its own philosophy, including the view that a person's posture reflects their mental, emotional, and spiritual state.

Yoga requires strength and flexibility; if you are lacking those, you will soon gain them if you perform the exercises regularly. Yoga exercises are meant to be performed as gentle stretching with a feeling of relaxation. According to yoga practitioners, if you are sore afterward, you are not doing it quite right.

Even though this is a very simple explanation of what yoga is, the primary benefit of practicing yoga for the average person is improved flexibility. Certainly, though, getting together with a group of people to be healthy and improve your posture will benefit your pursuit of better health.

If you're particularly stiff or immobile, starting with warm or hot yoga can relax your muscles more and help you benefit more from each class. As with anything that deals with your body and good health, consistency is important. Doing yoga once a year won't make much of a difference.

PILATES

Developed by Joseph Pilates, this exercise was designed to improve strength and flexibility without becoming "bulky." Pilates has enjoyed increased popularity with the more recent focus on improving one's "core." Pilates develops abdominal strength, improving your spinal support.

There are Pilates programs popping up everywhere, including home-study courses. Generally, there are two types: floor Pilates and classes utilizing reformers. Both are very beneficial.

As Pilates is another form of exercise, I hope you are starting to see that you are going to have to exercise to make an effective, lasting change to your posture.

► CHAPTER 9

HOW TO GET BETTER POSTURE FAST

We've covered how your posture forms, all the conditions that cause bad posture, underlying problems associated with bad posture, and the right way to have good posture in your daily life.

How do you get Better Posture Fast? How can you effect the greatest change in the shortest time possible? You've reached the part of the book that answers all of that for you.

Our mindset and our approach to achieving good posture is this: Let's make the tweaks to your activities that are causing the most damage, give you the right stretches and exercises that will make the greatest difference, give you recommendations for products that will actually help, and give you things you can do to keep it that way.

STEP 1

ALIGNMENT

EVALUATE YOUR DAILY ACTIVITIES

Starting with the basics, take a look at your main work activities. We primarily see patients that sit at computers all day, so that's an easy one. If your job doesn't require that you sit at a computer all day, look for the things you do repetitively or for extended periods. Are you balanced?

All your daily activities should provide some balance. That means you do as much for your front muscles as you do for your back muscles. You do as much for your right side as you do your left side.

Now, you're quickly going to realize this is impossible. You're going to have a dominant hand, and you're going to do way more "front" activities than "back" activities. Regardless, spend a day looking for the things you can change.

Can you raise your monitors? Can you move your monitors so that they are in front of you more than to the side? Are you sitting straight when you drive, or do you lean on the console? Do you always sit on the same spot on the couch?

You will not be able to perfectly balance everything, but look for anything that's way out of whack that can be changed and then make that change. We've provided different examples throughout the book of activities real patients had to change, so we hope that will help you as well.

Most activities that cause bad posture are things you do over and over again or things you do for long periods of time. Look for any of those and make the necessary modifications.

EVALUATE YOUR SLEEP POSTURE

If you're going to spend six to eight hours a night in a posture of some kind, let's make it as good as we can! If you're a stomach sleeper, you've got to start making a change. Find the right pillow and try sleeping on your side. Hug a body pillow to keep you as even and neutral as possible.

If you're a side sleeper, just make sure your pillow keeps your head neutral and that you've got a pillow between your knees. We still love the body pillow, but that's up to you.

If you're a back sleeper, get a pillow that has some neck support, and don't sleep on two pillows. Put a big pillow under your knees to help take some pressure off your lower back.

CONSIDER CHIROPRACTIC CARE

We say this as unbiased as we can, but you really should be seeing a chiropractor. There are so many advantages to being under regular chiropractic care, with better posture being just a small part.

Your nervous system controls everything in your whole body, which is why good posture is so important. Pressure on your nerves can affect many different aspects of your health, so it's important that you keep your nerves functioning as well as you can.

Also, movement in your spinal joints is what prevents you from developing degenerative changes. Areas of your spine that become stuck and out of place are the first to show signs of degeneration. Maintaining the function of your spinal joints will keep your spine healthy.

Not all chiropractors approach chiropractic care the same way. Some chiropractors are very sports-minded and do very little adjusting. They focus on exercise and on working on the soft tissues of the body. That's great, but that's not the kind of chiropractic care that will help you change your spine quite in the way we would recommend.

Some chiropractors focus entirely on auto-accident cases. Many of these offices also do very little adjusting to your spine. They are more focused on helping you heal from sprain/strain injuries and may have you do a bunch of passive therapies rather than perform chiropractic adjustments.

Unfortunately, there's no way of knowing which type of chiropractor you're going to see without doing a little research before you go. After we explain how we evaluate and care for our patients, we suggest that you find a chiropractic office reasonably close to you that does something similar to what we recommend.

Here's How We Evaluate and Treat Patients at Our Office (Which May Be Different Than Other Chiropractors You May See)

Throughout our careers, most of our new patients have come to us when they're in pain. Now we regularly see new patients that are not in a lot of pain, but are worried about bad posture and its potential long-term negative effects. Regardless of the reason someone first seeks out chiropractic care, the process in our office starts out the same way.

We start with an initial consultation to learn more about the patient, their goals, and why they decided to start chiropractic care. We are still surprised when new patients come to us and say they "just want to get popped" and aren't interested in reviewing their problem. "Something feels stuck," they say, adding they would like it to be quickly unstuck and don't want to hear anything else about it. While they may be right in their "assessment," we still want to talk about it first. Patients don't always understand some of the dangerous contraindications they may have that will prevent them getting safely adjusted.

Next, we do an examination, which starts with a posture

evaluation, much like the one we described in the book. We then check the spine's range of motion and use our hands to feel along the spine for areas of dysfunction. We can tell which spinal segments are moving well and which are not simply by feeling them and doing small pushes to test how they move.

We perform orthopedic and neurological tests that are standard tests for all chiropractors and medical doctors. Each orthopedic test is designed to check on a specific joint or rule out a specific condition. The neurological tests give us a better idea as to how the nervous system is functioning and if the condition requires an immediate referral to a different provider.

The next step is to take any necessary X-rays. We primarily do spinal X-rays, but sometimes a patient's case requires an X-ray of a joint in the arm or leg. Once the X-rays are completed, we use special software to analyze them and take measurements. The software pulls up the X-ray image and allows us to draw lines all over it, utilizing bony landmarks in the vertebrae as guides. These measurements are key to the results we see with our patients, as we use this information to guide our adjustments and to verify our results.

From these lines, we come up with a one-page document that tells the chiropractor what was on the patient's X-rays. The chiropractor refers to this document on each of the visits so they know which bones need to be adjusted and in which direction. This means each visit will consistently move the spine in the right direction.

Our office has several chiropractors on staff, so the adjustments patients receive from one doctor will be consistent with any other doctor that performs the adjustment on that visit (*if your regular doctor happens to be out of the office that day*). This also avoids the issue that can come up when a patient says, "Whatever you did last time worked, so please do it again," and the chiropractor doesn't know what was done on the previous visit. We know what we did last time!

It's the analysis and then the consistency in the execution of the plan that allows for a consistent result. Unfortunately, there are chiropractors out there (*and patients*) that are happy just to hear some things crack without consideration of moving the bones consistently in the proper direction.

The "cracks" release endorphins and provide short-term pain relief. It just feels good to get adjusted, but it's about more than that. We want for the adjustment to feel good, but we adjust you in a specific way so you won't need to get adjusted as often to stay in proper alignment. Our patients tend start off on treatment plans that recommend they come in more frequently at first, but then less and less often as they improve.

We continue to give our patients recommendations throughout their care, but most patients graduate to a "wellness" adjustment where they come in periodically to undo anything that's happened since the last visit. (*Since almost everyone just goes back to the same activities they were doing before they came to our office.*)

Patients can still see significant improvement in their posture without chiropractic care, but they will get there a lot faster with chiropractic adjustments. If for some reason you've had a bad experience with a chiropractor in the past, don't give up on all chiropractors. Find someone that will listen to your concerns and adapt their adjusting style to accommodate your preferences.

UTILIZE A NECK WEDGE

If you've not used a neck wedge, you've been missing out! If you've begun to lose the normal curve of your neck and have forward-head posture, you'll love using the neck wedge. It's an inexpensive foam triangle that helps improve your neck curve.

Ideally, your neck has a curve of thirty-five degrees. The best patient success story we've seen is a patient who went from a negative twenty-five (-25) degree curve to a positive two-degree curve in just a few months. Even better, his forward-head posture changed substantially during that time. He was consistent with his chiropractic care, but he used his neck wedge every day.

The neck wedge is more practical and useful than a lot of the posture gadgets we see for neck traction online, plus, as we mentioned, it's inexpensive. Using it consistently is the biggest factor in its success. Using it occasionally won't change the curve of your neck much, particularly if you're spending ten to twelve hours on your computer and phone all day.

For a video demonstration and more information about the neck wedge, visit https://www.betterposturefast.com/step1.

MAKE CHANGES TO YOUR LUMBAR CURVE

It's possible to change the curve in your lower back, but the tricky part is knowing if you have too much or not enough curve. This cannot be determined easily without an X-ray. If you know for sure how much curve you have in your lower back, you can get started. If you have any doubt, we recommend waiting to do anything until you get an X-ray of the area.

If you need more curve, utilizing a rolled-up towel (*or some other roll*) under your lower back while you lie on your neck wedge will help. If you have too much curve, then you need to lie on your back with your knees bent and try to pull your belly button down to the floor.

For a video demonstration and more information about increasing or decreasing your lower-back curve, visit https://www. betterposturefast.com/step1. In the video we share on that page, we also show you some inexpensive rolls you can purchase to help the lumbar curve.

ORTHOTICS

To what extent does the alignment of your feet affect your posture? More than you'd think. Since most of our patients sit all day, we've found that most changes occur using the other recommendations in this book. However, special custom shoe inserts called orthotics are still a good idea.

The most common change that occurs in our patients' feet is the rolling in of the feet and ankles. This creates instability in the knees, hips … and all the way up the spine.

The orthotics we recommend stabilize the foot and keep the foot from rolling in. Some orthotics are very rigid, and we've found that our patients just can't wear them for long periods of time.

There are several orthotic options out there, including seeing a podiatrist for their recommendations. The biggest difference between orthotics at our office and orthotics with a podiatrist is how the foot is analyzed.

Podiatrists measure the foot in a non-weight-bearing position (*up in the air*), while all our analyses are done in a weight-bearing position. The same concept applies to us when we take X-rays. Most X-rays at medical offices are done with the patient lying down, but we have the patient stand to see how gravity affects the spine.

Both styles of orthotics have been shown to be effective, but we believe that weight-bearing analysis is better. For more information about orthotics and our recommendations, visit https://www.betterposturefast.com/step1.

STEP 2

EXERCISES

It is important that you understand that your simple, boring daily activities created your bad-posture problems in the first place, and that you need to do the exercises outlined here to counteract your normal daily activities. These exercises do not need to be complicated to work incredibly well.

Give the exercises a consistent effort. When done daily, you should begin to notice in just a few days a difference in your ability to stand up straight, and your pain and discomfort should begin to fade. Do these exercises every day for a month, and you will be amazed by the difference in your posture.

Some people still think that just because they work out all the time, they don't need exercises as uncomplicated as these. We could go to the gym right now and find people in great shape and full of muscles who have horrible posture. What are they missing from their exercise regimen? Take a look at the exercises listed here for your answer.

As always, should you experience pain (*particularly sharp pain*) …
STOP! Some soreness is okay and is to be expected when you start any exercise program. If you are very sore, you should back off the repetitions or the frequency of the exercises.

If you have further questions, please consult with your healthcare professional.

Each exercise is an intense focus on a small area. Focus on that area with each repetition, and relax as you return to the neutral (*starting*) position.

The goal of these exercises is to balance out the front, side, and back muscles, so keep that in mind when doing them. Also, don't just do the ones you like if they aren't addressing all sides of your body.

Soon you will see that your weaker areas are getting stronger. As you strengthen all areas, you should strive to develop all areas equally. This is the key to balance and to good posture.

Also, if over time the number of repetitions becomes too easy, it's okay to do more! If you're going to continue to strengthen your muscles, you'll need to continue to challenge them!

Our goal isn't to overwhelm you with a bunch of exercises that you can't do easily or consistently. If you can commit to fifteen minutes a day, you will be light-years ahead of the bad-posture direction you were headed.

The point of most of these exercises is to build strength where the weak muscle is not supporting you properly and to stretch areas that are too tight from your daily activities.

Pick the region of the body that is giving you the most trouble and start there.

Try each exercise a few times before giving up. Depending on how weak or deconditioned a particular muscle is, you may find that you have trouble doing the movement at all. As long as you're not experiencing pain while doing the movement, you should be able to continue.

Video demonstrations for all of these exercises is available on our website at https://www.betterposturefast.com/step2.

NECK EXERCISES

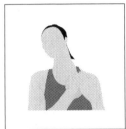

Anterior Neck Stretch

Stretch the front of your neck, look up and over your shoulder – hold for 10 seconds and then repeat on each side at least 2 times.

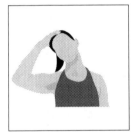

Side Neck Stretch

Bring ear to shoulder – hold for 10 seconds on each side. Repeat 2 – 3 times per session.

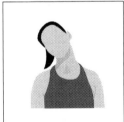

Trapezius and Neck Release

Bring the arm that is on the same side you'll be stretching behind your back. This will increase the intensity of the stretch.

Hold it in place taking deep breaths. Hold for 30 seconds and then switch to the other side.

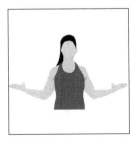

Neck Stretch Using Shoulder Rotation

Bend your elbows at 90 degrees and then pull your arms back, concentrating on bringing your shoulder blades together. Open up your chest (*and optionally, lean your head back to open up more of your neck*).

Hold and stretch back, taking a deep breath. Repeat 10 times.

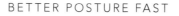
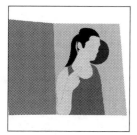

Neck Exercises Using a Ball

You want to strengthen the neck in all directions, so plan on doing front, back, and both sides. The ball is there to give you something to push into, and to provide a little resistance.

Start with ball behind you, pushing in isometrically and relax. Repeat 10 times. Then move into flexion and extension. Repeat 10 times. Look left and right while pushing your head into the ball. Repeat 10 times. Last, do a "W" motion, repeat 3 times.

Move to the side of your neck. Pushing into the ball, then looking front and back, then looking into and away from the wall. Repeat 10 times each movement.

Move to the front of your neck. Repeat the same motions and when the ball was in the back. Contract, then flexion/extension, then looking left/right and ending with the "W."

Move to the other side of your neck and do the same movements as done for the previous side.

Last, work on your cervical curve with the ball at the back of your neck and contract and stretch the front of your body. Repeat 10 times.

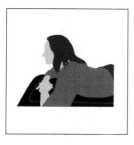

Neck Extensions

Start face down on your bed or the floor. You'll be using the weight of your head to strengthen the back of your neck. Put your face down and raise only your head as far back as you can comfortably go. Repeat 10 times for 3 sets.

For a video demonstration of each neck exercise, visit https://www.betterposturefast.com/step2.

SHOULDER EXERCISES

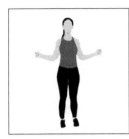

Shoulder Squeezes

Relax head and neck and stand with good posture. Squeeze your shoulders back and avoid shrugging the shoulders and keep the abdominal region tight. Hold for 5 seconds.

Relax the shoulders.
Perform 2 sets of 12 - 15 repetitions.

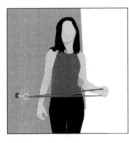

External Rotation Exercise for the Shoulder

Attach a resistance band to a stable object at waist level (*ex. Door knob, bed post, dresser drawer, etc.*) Roll shoulders back and down and maintain this position

Place a towel between the elbow and side of the body, then slowly rotate your hand away from the abdomen while keeping the shoulder still.

Hold for 3 seconds. Perform 2 sets of 12-15 repetitions.

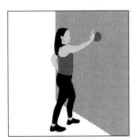

Physio ball Scapular Exercise

Stand with hand placed on physio ball (*any ball will work*) against a wall.

Move the arm in a clockwise motion slowly for 30 seconds and then move the arm in a counter-clockwise motion for 30 seconds

Maintain shoulders back and down. Do your best to perform 2 sets of the exercise

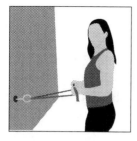

Horizontal Rows

Secure the resistance band around a stable object, like a door knob or bed post. While standing grab both sides of the resistance band and bring shoulders back and down

With arms extended, slowly pull hands straight back until they are even with your body

Pinch the shoulder blades together and hold 3 seconds. Perform 2 sets of 12 - 15 repetitions.

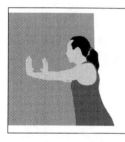

Scapula Retractions

Stand near a wall and place your hands on the wall in front of you. Concentrate on squeezing your shoulder blades together, like you're trying to squeeze an orange between them.

Perform 2 sets of 15 repetitions.

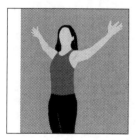

Wall Angels

Stand against a wall with arms by your side.

Keeping elbows to the side, slowly raise your arms above your head while keeping them against the wall. Hold for 3 seconds and slowly slide arms down. Imagine putting your elbows into your back pockets and squeeze your shoulder blades together on the way down.

Perform 2 sets of 12 - 15 repetitions.

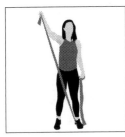

Shoulder Diagonals (Y)

Patient stands with the resistance band under their opposite foot, while grasping the resistance band. Bring your shoulders back and down.

With your hand at your opposite hip, slowly raise it up across your body, as if you are drawing a sword from its sheath.

Hold 3 seconds and repeat 12 - 15 times for each shoulder.

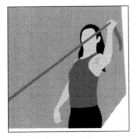

External Rotations at 90 Degrees

Attach a resistance band to a stable object at shoulder level (*ex. Door knob, bed post, dresser drawer, etc.*). Grab the resistance band with your palm facing down to the floors and arm at shoulder level and slowly rotate hand back and behind the body.

Hold for 3 seconds. Perform 2 sets of 10 - 12 repetitions.

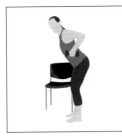

Bent-Over Rows

With a dumbbell in each hand, bend over at about a 45-degree angle (*no further*). Keep the back straight throughout the exercise. Brace your abdominals and breathe in.

Lift the weights straight up, exhaling. While lifting, the arms should go no higher than parallel with the shoulders - slightly lower than the shoulders is fine. While lifting, try to keep the wrists from excessive extra movement down or to the side. Do not squat down and up after the initial pose. No movement of the legs occurs throughout the exercise.

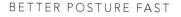
Lower the weights in a controlled manner while inhaling. Remain bent over until all repetitions are complete. Perform 2 sets of 10 - 12 repetitions.

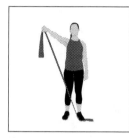

Scaptions

Stand on one end to secure the band. Grasp the band at your side with the thumb up.

Lift the band slightly in front of your side at 30 degrees in front of the body while keeping the elbow straight.

Hold for a count of 2 and slowly return. Perform 2 sets of 10 - 12 repetitions.

For a video demonstration of each shoulder exercise, visit https://www.betterposturefast.com/step2.

MID BACK EXERCISES

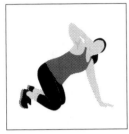

Kneeling T-Spine Rotations

Start in a kneeling position on the floor with your back in a neutral position and your hands right above your shoulders. Reach through your opposite arm and leg and try to feel a stretch on the back of your shoulder and mid back. Pull your arm back and open your chest up in to a fly position trying to feel a stretch on the front of your shoulder and lower back.

Perform 2 sets of 10 repetitions on each side.

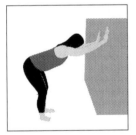

Half Wall Hang

Stand facing a wall and then place your hands on the wall as you walk your feet back and move your hands down the wall until your chest is parallel to the ground.

Walk your feet back and set your hands up on the wall so that you are bending at the hips to about 90 degrees and your legs are straight.

Hang over with your hands on the wall, try to extend your back with your arms straight and your biceps by your ears. Try to extend your spine and create a nice straight line from your hands on the wall to your tailbone.

Press your chest out toward the ground as you extend your spine. Drive your chest through your arms and feel a nice stretch through your lats and triceps.

Hold for 20 - 30 seconds and breathe and focus on extending your thoracic spine as you keep your abdominal area engaged so you do not hyperextend the lower back.

Repeat 5 times.

***Beginners may need to start with their hands higher up on the wall and their feet closer in so that they are not leaning over too much.*

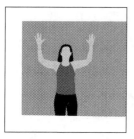

Wall Slides

Lean your back against the wall with your feet a few inches from the wall. Bend your knees slightly and press your back into the wall. Try to keep the lower back flat against the wall throughout the movement. Do not arch the lower back.

Press your upper back into the wall and relax your head against the wall as you bend your arms and place the back of your hands against the wall right at each side of your head. Keeping your back firmly against the wall and your abdomen tight, slide the back of your hands up the wall as far as possible. Then slowly slide them back down.

Do not slide them up further if your lower back is coming away from the wall and you are getting the extension from your lower back instead of your upper back.

Repeat 10 times reaching up the wall and each time try to get higher up the wall. Perform 2 sets.

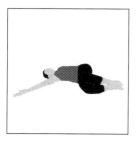

Side Lying Rotations

Lie on your side on the floor with the knees bent to 90 degrees.

Place the arms out in front of you with the palms facing each other. Slowly slide the top hand over the bottom arm toward your chest and across to the shoulder.

PHILIP V. CORDOVA, D.C. & NATALIE A. CORDOVA, D.C.

Allow the trunk to rotate and slowly extend the arm from the shoulder and then the elbow, reaching out with the fingertips and turning the head to look down the line of the arm. Make sure the pelvis and hips are still pointing forward.

Reverse this sequence and finish by sliding the palm of the top hand beyond the bottom hand. Repeat slowly and continuously 5 times then roll over and repeat on the other side.

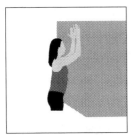

Elbow Slides on the Wall

Stand facing a wall and then place your elbows on the wall as you walk your feet back.

You are in a plank position while up against the wall. Slowly slide your elbows up the wall as you engage your core. Maintain a strong spine and abdominal muscles as you reach your elbows as high up the wall without bending the spine.

The focus of the movement is between the arm and the upper body. Pause. Then lower your elbows to the lower, plank position. Repeat 10 times for 2 sets.

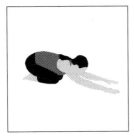

Child's Pose with Movement

Start on your hands and knees. Bring your knees and feet together as you sit your butt back on your heels and stretch your arms forward. Allow the upper back to stretch and pull away from your lower back.

Walk your hands as far to the right as you can. Breathe deep and then relax. Hold for 3 – 4 breaths and then walk your hands to the left. Hold again for 3 – 4 breaths. Walk your hands back to center and then sit up. Repeat 2 more times.

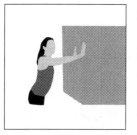

Scapula Push-Ups

Face a wall, standing 2 feet away. Place hands on the wall. Lower your chest toward the wall without bending the elbows. As you approach the wall, your shoulder blades should feel like they are going away from the wall as your ribs are going toward the wall. Aim for a large gap between the ribs and the shoulder blades. Return to the starting position and repeat. Perform 2 sets of 10 repetitions.

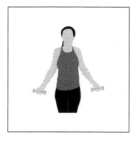

Trap Activations

Stand with a light weight in your hands. Arms should be to the side with your palms facing away. Shrug your shoulders, focusing on contracting your upper back (trapezius muscles). Hold for 3 seconds and then relax and lower your shoulders. Perform 2 sets of 10 repetitions.

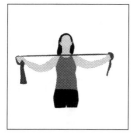

Pull Aparts

Standing with feet shoulder width apart, grab the handles of the resistance band with each hand, then loop the band once or twice more around each hand to desired tightness. Holding hands straight out in front of you at shoulder height, pull the band open as arms go out to the sides and band comes in towards chest. Keep your shoulders back at all times.

Slowly release hands back to start position and repeat. Perform 2 sets of 12 - 15 repetitions.

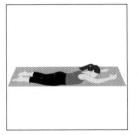

Superman

Lay face down on a mat or flat surface, with your arm outstretched. Keep your hands and arms straight throughout the entire exercise. Raise your arms and legs 4 – 5 inches off the ground. Hold for 5 seconds, then return to the starting position. Repeat 10 times. Perform 2 sets.

For a video demonstration of each of the mid back exercises, visit https://www.betterposturefast.com/step2.

LOW BACK EXERCISES

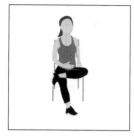

Hip-Rotator Stretch – Static

Sit in a chair with one leg on the floor. Bend the other leg so that your ankle rests on top of your first leg's knee. Bend at the hip, feeling the stretch in the back of the hip that is in the up position. Hold for 2 minutes and then switch sides. Hold the other side for 2 minutes (at least).

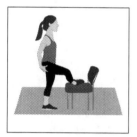

Modified Pigeon Pose

Stand on one leg. The other leg is flexed and the ankle should be turned in so that you can rest the lower leg on a box or a chair. Bend at the hip, stretching the back of the hip. Hold for 2 minutes, then switch sides. Hold other side for 2 minutes.

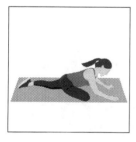

Pigeon Pose

Start in a plank stance. Bend one knee and bring it forward to the same elbow. Turn the knee so the lower leg crosses the body like a "T." Lower the upper body, which should be bending at the hips and stretch the back of the hip. The other leg stays extended behind the body. Hold for 2 minutes and then switch sides. Hold the other side for 2 minutes.

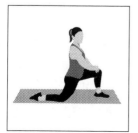

Hip-Flexor Stretch – Static

Lunge forward with the front knee bent and the back leg extended behind you. Lower the back leg a couple of inches so that you feel the stretch in the front of the hip. (*Increase intensity by bringing the knee to the floor.*) Hold onto a chair for balance, if needed.

The stretch should be felt in the extended leg at the front of the hip. Hold for 2 minutes and then switch sides. Hold other side for 2 minutes.

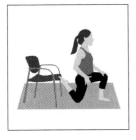

Couch Stretch

Bend the knee of the leg you are stretching so that the knee is on the ground (*or on a pillow*) and the foot is propped up against a wall (*or the couch*). Lunge forward with the other knee bent, but don't bend it beyond the foot that is planted on the ground.

Hold onto a chair for balance, if needed. The stretch should be felt in the back of the leg and at the front of the hip. Aim to straighten your upper body in line with the leg that's parallel to the wall. Hold for 2 minutes and then switch sides. Hold the other side for an additional 2 minutes.

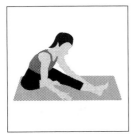

Hamstring Stretch – Static

Sit on the floor with your leg stretched out in front of you. You can fold the other leg in towards you. Bend at the hip, reaching for your toes. You are lengthening the portion or your hamstring that crosses the back of the knee. Hold this for 2 minutes and then switch sides. Hold the other side for 2 minutes.

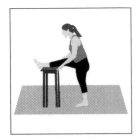

Standing Hamstring Stretch

Stand on one leg, with the other leg extended onto the back of a sturdy chair or surface. Band at the hip, reaching for your toes. You are lengthening the hamstring as it crosses the

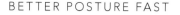

back of the knee. Hold this for 2 minutes and then switch sides. Hold the other side for 2 minutes.

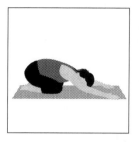

Child's Pose

Start on your hands and knees. Bring your knees and feet together as you sit your butt onto your heels. Stretch your arms forward and allow the upper back to stretch and pull away from the lower back. Breathe in deep and then relax. Hold for 8 – 10 breaths and then sit up. Repeat 2 more times.

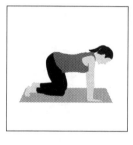

Cat/Cow Stretch

Start on all fours and then place your wrists underneath your shoulders with your knees underneath your hips. Balance your weight evenly between all four points. Inhale as you look up and let your stomach drop down toward the mat.

Exhale as you tuck your chin into your chest, draw your navel toward your spine, and arch your spine toward the ceiling. Maintain awareness of your body as you do this movement. Focus on squeezing and releasing tension in your body. Continue this fluid movement for 30 seconds to 1 minute.

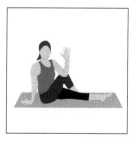

Seated Spinal Twist

From a seated position, keep your left leg straight and bend your right leg so your foot is flat. Place your right hand on the floor behind you for support, like a tripod, and twist so you can hook your left elbow over the right thigh.

If this is too much, you can also grab hold of your right knee and twist to look over your right shoulder. Lengthen your spine as you twist your body to the right. Try to keep your hips square to deepen the twist in your spine. Turn your gaze to look over either shoulder. Hold this pose for up to 1 minute. Repeat on the other side.

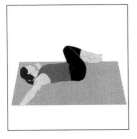

Two-Knee Spinal Twist

Lie on your back with your knees drawn into your chest and your arms extended to the side. Slowly lower your legs to the left side while keeping your knees as close together as possible. You may place a pillow under both knees or in between your knees. You can use your left hand to gently press down on your knees.

Focus on breathing deeply in this position. Hold this pose for at least 30 seconds. Repeat on the opposite side. Modify by lengthening the leg you are not crossing over the body to get the knee that you are stretching further away and therefore a deeper stretch.

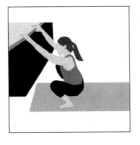

Deep Squat Stretch

Hold onto a counter while standing with your feet shoulder width apart. Lower into a deep squat, pushing your knee out. Hold in the bottom of the squat for 3 seconds, flexing the lower spine. Perform 10 repetitions, then hold in a deep squat position for 5 deep breaths.

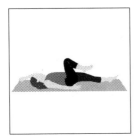

Cross/Crawl

This brain and posture training exercise can most easily be done in a supine position (*laying on your back*). Put both legs straight and place both arms down at the sides. This technique may also be done standing or sitting. Raise and elevate the right arm above the head, at the same time raise the opposite leg, bending the knee.

Improve your results by turning the head towards the raised right arm, then straighten your head as the arm and left leg come down. Repeat procedure with left arm & opposite right leg, turning head towards the raised left arm. Breathe in as the opposite arm and leg raise, exhale as the arm and leg come down. Do in series of 12 right and 12 left for a total of 24 movements. Visualize marching.

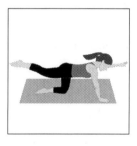

Bird Dog

Kneel with knees hip-width apart and your hands placed on the ground shoulder-width apart. Hold your core/abdominal muscles tight and strong. Practice lifting one hand and the opposite knee just an inch or two off the floor while balancing on the other hand and knee and keeping your weight centered. Continue to point the arm out straight in front and extend the opposite leg behind you.

You should form one straight line from your hand to your foot, keeping hips squared to the ground. If your low back begins to sag, raise your leg only as high as you can while keeping your back straight. Hold for a few seconds then return your hands and knees to the starting position. Keep your abs engaged throughout the entire exercise, and work to minimize any extra motion in your hips during the weight shift.

Aim to complete 5 strong repetitions on each side, 10 repetitions in total. Add additional sets as you feel comfortable, up to 3 sets.

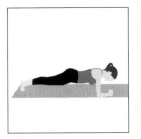

Plank

Place forearms on the floor with elbows aligned below shoulders and arms parallel to your body at about shoulder width. If flat palms bother your wrists, clasp your hands together. Ground toes into the floor and squeeze glutes to stabilize your body. Your legs should be working, too — be careful not to lock or hyperextend your knees.

Neutralize your neck and spine by looking at a spot on the floor about a foot beyond your hands. Your head should be in line with your back. Hold the position for 20 seconds. As you get more comfortable with the move, hold your plank for as long as possible without compromising your form or breath

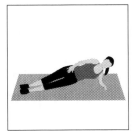

Side Plank

Get into a side plank position. Drop your bottom hip toward the floor. Reverse the movement and lift hip up as high as you can. Repeat 10 times. Repeat on the other side.

Modified: do this up against a wall on your elbow. Feet parallel to the wall and about a foot away from your upper body. Move your hip toward the wall and then back to your starting position. Repeat 10 times. Repeat on the other side.

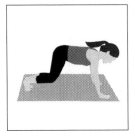

Quad Plank

Start on all fours and raise your knees off the ground. Arch your back, raise the upper body up, opening the lower back. Hold for 20 – 30 seconds.

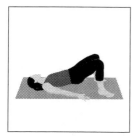

Glute Bridge

Lie on your back with your knees bent and your feet flat on the floor hip-width apart. Your arms should be relaxed at your sides. Lift your glutes off the floor, tucking your pelvis to flatten out your lower back, pushing with your heels. Your body should look like a straight line from your knees to your shoulders. Squeeze your glutes and abdominals, hold for 2 seconds, and then take 3 seconds to slowly lower your back to the starting position. Perform 3 sets of 10 repetitions.

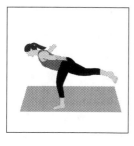

Single-Leg Deadlift

Stand with both feet under hips. Shift your weight to the right leg, which should be straight with a slight bend in the knee. Begin to lift your left foot back behind you, keeping your leg straight. Simultaneously, slowly start hinging at the waist, tipping your torso forward until it's almost parallel to the floor. Keep your arms straight, at shoulder height, and perpendicular to the floor at all times.

At the bottom of the position, your body should be in a straight line from the top of your head to the bottom of your left foot. Hold for 3 sec. Then, begin pulling your left leg forward while keeping it straight, and lift your torso up until you're standing again. Repeat all reps on one side, then switch legs.

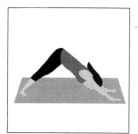

Downward-Facing Dog

Get on all fours. Place your hands in alignment under your wrists and your knees under your hips. Press into your hands, tuck your toes under, and lift up your knees. Bring your sit bones up toward the ceiling. Keep a slight bend in your knees and lengthen your spine and tailbone. Keep your heels slightly off the ground. Press firmly into your hands.

Distribute your weight evenly between both sides of your body, paying attention to the position of your hips and shoulders. Keep your head in line with your upper arms or with your chin tucked in slightly. Hold this pose for 30 sec-1min

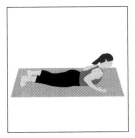

Cobra Pose

Lie on your stomach with your hands under your shoulders and your fingers facing forward. Don't allow your elbows to go out to the side. Press into your hands to slowly lift your head, chest, and shoulders. You can lift partway, halfway, or all the way up. Don't go to the point of pain.

Maintain a slight bend in your elbows. You can let your head drop back. Release back down to your mat on an exhale. Look straight ahead or slightly upward as you lengthen the back of your neck. Remain in this pose for up to 1 minute. Rest before repeating the pose.

For a video demonstration of each low back exercise, visit https://www.betterposturefast.com/step2.

STEP 3

MOBILITY

You've worked on alignment, you've been doing exercises and stretches, so why do you need to work on mobility? Unfortunately, our bodies get stuck in positions we do all the time, and we've had injuries that have created scar tissue and "knots" in our muscles.

We know you've felt them, and they're holding you back from becoming truly flexible and functional. Mobility is one of those things that a lot of people don't like to address at first, but later they wonder how they ever got by without it. It's a "hurts so good" kind of activity.

Mobility exercises can hurt – but within reason; they shouldn't hurt the entire time you're doing them. If you feel like the exercise is not getting any easier, we've provided some options. If you feel like the device should be firmer or more challenging, we've got you covered there too.

When we ask patients to make a change for their posture, they usually implement only a couple things. They'll adjust their computer monitor, and they'll do a few stretches. Some people will occasionally mix in an exercise here or there. Almost everyone fights us on mobility work, and it can have the greatest impact. Working on your mobility gives you the most "bang for your buck" when it comes to time spent on a home-exercise program, so give it a try!

FOAM ROLLER

It's really much easier to show you how to use a foam roller in a video, so we've put that together for you if you visit https://www.betterposturefast.com/step3.

The general rule for foam rolling your back is to lie on the floor, place the foam roller perpendicular to your spine, and roll back and forth on it. Start at the upper back and stop before you get to the lower back. Some people can roll their lower back, but for most people, this seems to cause more pain and isn't worth it.

To increase the intensity of rolling in the upper- and mid-back areas, try reaching overhead or giving yourself a hug while using the foam roller.

For foam rolling other areas of the body, you'll likely still need to be on the floor. It will take some practice, but you'll find ways to get the area of the body you want to work onto the foam roller. You'll figure out how to place your body in a position that will enable you to put some pressure on that area, even if it feels a bit awkward at first.

The video on the "Step 3" page of our website gives you a basic routine that will help you use your foam roller on as much of your body as possible. If you want help finding softer or firmer foam rollers, we've got some options for you there as well.

LACROSSE BALL OR "PEANUT"

When doing mobility work, you'll find that your body has many different "nooks and crannies" that the foam roller can't reach. You'll need something smaller to apply specific pressure to a knot or other small area of complaint.

A tennis ball works for some people, but you'll need something firmer to work on that knot. In our home, we keep a lacrosse ball, a baseball, and a softball available and ready for use. The lacrosse ball is the most popular and can be picked up for a few dollars at our office or any local sporting-goods store.

When using a ball for mobility, you want to think of it more like an elbow. You don't want to roll around on it, but rather use it in one spot at a time and apply continuous pressure. Rolling around on the knot tends to irritate it rather than break it up.

Lie on the floor or use a wall to brace yourself and then place the ball where you want to work. Apply pressure for five to ten seconds, and then move to another spot. You'll find that some spots need a baseball, while others need a different ball. Experiment with them and see which one works best for you.

How long you use the ball each session is up to you. You will eventually feel the knot start to go away, and that's all you need for that session. You can do this type of mobility work often, but if you find that you're getting too sore, be sure to give yourself a break. You can overdo it!

A "peanut" is two lacrosse balls taped together to make a peanut shape. This is particularly useful when working on your middle-back area. The spine fits neatly between the two lacrosse balls, so most of the pressure is on the muscles on either side of the spine. Again, don't roll the peanut; just apply pressure, then move to a new area and apply pressure again.

MASSAGER

Massagers are very popular right now, especially those that are more percussion-oriented and not just vibrational. The "hitting" of the percussion massager does a great job of working out knots, increasing circulation, and relaxing the muscles.

They can be hundreds of dollars, so many patients still choose to stick with the cheaper lacrosse-ball option. However, we've found the cost of the massager to be well worth the investment and time spent using it.

For a list of recommended massagers, visit https://www.better posturefast.com/step3.

► CHAPTER 10

NOW WHAT? WHAT SHOULD YOU DO NEXT?

Congratulations on finishing the book! Now you know way more about improving your posture than you ever thought you would. It's time to take some action to have Better Posture Fast. You can do it!

Regardless of your age, the process to improve your posture is the same. Age (*but more importantly, how much damage you have in your spine*) does play a part in how long it will take to improve your posture, but you can improve it no matter how bad it is.

Too many patients confuse "perfect posture" with "better posture." You may not be able to achieve perfect posture after a certain age or once degeneration has crept into your spine, but you can make changes that improve your health, increase movement, and decrease or eliminate pain.

The path to improving your posture on your own is to follow the three steps we outlined above.

Step 1: Work on alignment. Use some of the recommended devices and watch your daily activities for areas of imbalance. It's not just your computer that will need to be adjusted. Be mindful of what you're doing repeatedly or for extended periods of time and see how you're doing.

Step 2: Exercise! For some reason people think this means "do more walking." That's not what we're saying. Start with the neck and mid-back exercises. You will see the most change by doing these exercises consistently.

Step 3: Do mobility work. Get a foam roller and a lacrosse ball and spend fifteen minutes a few times a week finding knots or areas of restriction and get after them. The foam roller covers the most ground, but the lacrosse ball is also very helpful – so get both.

If you want to speed up this whole process even further, we recommend getting to a chiropractor as soon as possible! We explained our process and approach earlier in the book, and we do recommend that you go to a chiropractor that will evaluate your spine with X-rays.

There are many adjusting techniques out there, so find the one that works best for you. However, the way the analysis is done and the method by which your progress will be measured are important considerations. Finding the least expensive chiropractor may sound like a good idea, but not at the risk of a bad initial analysis.

Take action, and you will have Better Posture Fast.

ADDITIONAL INFORMATION & RESOURCES

We have more to share with you, and we will keep updating our website and adding more information to it whenever necessary. We review other books and posture gadgets as they become available and will add new exercises that we find are helping our patients the most.

Get on our newsletter list by visiting our website at https://www.betterposturefast.com and get additional resources at https://www.betterposturefast.com/resources.

Reach out to us on our website or via social media:

Facebook: https://www.facebook.com/betterposturefast
Instagram: @betterposturefast

We check and respond to all questions as quickly as we can because we want to help you achieve better posture and good health!

ABOUT THE AUTHORS

Drs. Philip and Natalie Cordova met at Parker College of Chiropractic in Dallas, Texas and got married the day after they graduated in December 1996. After initially practicing in Phoenix, Arizona, they moved to Houston, Texas in 2000.

While raising 3 sons and building their chiropractic practice, Dr. Natalie Cordova created a posture exercise DVD called Posture Confidence. Promoting this exercise program became a passion for Dr. Philip Cordova, who created a website and started selling this DVD all over the world. Later, they co-wrote a book with the same title.

They currently have 2 offices in Houston, Texas and love sharing tips and exercises on improving posture with their patients. After creating hundreds of videos and blog posts, they decided it was time to put all of the information together in one place to help people achieve Better Posture Fast.

They are both still currently in active chiropractic practice. They enjoy exercising (*running, yoga, and CrossFit*) and spending time with their family.

Printed in the United States
by Baker & Taylor Publisher Services